THE SODIUM COUNTER

BY
WILLIAM I. KAUFMAN

BERKLEY BOOKS, NEW YORK

THE SODIUM COUNTER

A Berkley Book/published by arrangement with
the author

PRINTING HISTORY
Jove edition/February 1984
Berkley edition/February 1986

ISBN: 0-425-08779-4

Berkley books are published by The Berkley Publishing Group,
200 Madison Avenue, New York, NY 10016.
The name "BERKLEY" and the stylized "B" with design
are trademarks belonging to Berkley Publishing Corporation.

PRINTED IN THE UNITED STATES OF AMERICA

CONTENTS

Acknowledgment

All medical information in the Introduction was either provided by or supervised by David Edelbaum, M.D., F.A.C.P.

I am grateful to Dr. Edelbaum for his guidance.

INTRODUCTION

While everyone is aware of the ravages of alcohol, drugs, and too much food, we have only recently become aware of the dangers of too great a salt intake. "Killer salt" and "saltaholic" are terms that are used more and more in our everyday vocabulary. A large percentage of the deaths in this country are related to cardiovascular-circulatory causes, and hypertension (high blood pressure) contributes to most of these in some way. More than 20% of all Americans suffer from hypertension which, unlike cancer or diabetes, is referred to as "the silent killer." The leading contributor to this disease is salt.

Many studies from all over the world have shown that the amount of salt consumed by a person is directly related to the incidence of high blood pressure and the complications of high blood pressure, such as stroke, heart disease, and kidney failure. Take, for example, northern Japan. On the average, each inhabitant of that part of the country consumes about 6 teaspoons of salt a day. The death rate due to stroke and complications of hypertension is staggeringly high. In fact, in some areas, half of the population have high blood pressure.

The Nutrition Board of the National Research Council suggests that the average adult should use no more than ½ to 1 teaspoon of salt a day. Yet the average American consumes about 2 to 2½ teaspoons a day. This is approximately 5,000 mg of sodium, which is over twenty times more than what the body needs.

5

In the presence of normal kidney function, any intake of salt above 200 to 250 mg a day is excreted. Conversely, if a person with normal kidneys were to follow an absolutely salt-free diet, the body would excrete virtually no salt after a few days. While many people suffer no apparent ill effects from an excess of salt, there is now evidence to suggest that for people with a tendency toward high blood pressure excessive salt intake can spell trouble—especially if you are Black.

While it is very difficult to determine in advance who is and who is not excessively sensitive to salt, medical opinion suggests that everyone will benefit from a reasonable modification of salt intake. Interestingly enough, blood pressure can be dropped as much as 10% by a one-third reduction in salt intake. If you have high blood pressure and take medication, the effect of the medication may be partially or completely negated by high salt consumption, so that the restriction of dietary sodium is an extremely important aspect of high blood pressure treatment.

How can the salt problem be eliminated and how can you reduce your salt intake? One good way is to use *The Sodium Counter*.

Even if you give up using salt at the table and cut down on the salt you use in cooking, you will not completely solve your salt intake problem. Neither will it be solved by giving up salted pretzels, sour pickles, and sauerkraut. The real problem is that salt is found in almost all of America's favorite foods and in virtually all processed food. The sodium in baking powder and baking soda makes cereals and baked goods major carriers in the salt war. Because of the growing popularity of frozen and processed foods, which are loaded

6

with the most effective preservative, salt, and because of the new American tendency to dine out, most Americans and many people all over the world are ingesting relatively high quantities of salt.

Please bear in mind that I recommend cutting down your salt intake but not cutting out salt completely. The necessity for controlling your intake of salt should be discussed with your doctor before you consider modifying your habit. Only your physician can tell you how much salt you should consume. If your doctor advises you to reduce your salt intake, his or her instructions will be easier to follow if you use *The Sodium Counter*.

Sodium is an extremely important element and an adequate level of sodium is necessary to maintain the normal functions of the body. Under certain conditions, too little salt can result in serious medical problems. This usually occurs in situations where there is an underlying kidney disease so that the kidney cannot properly conserve salt (one of its main functions) or where people are taking diuretics for a variety of reasons.

Since many people who are on low sodium diets are also taking diuretics, I have included the milligram count for potassium because it is essential that people on diuretics also monitor their potassium intake. For these people, the proper level of potassium must be carefully maintained for normal body functioning. The average person needs about 2,500 mg of potassium each day.

Sodium and potassium mg counts listed are based on information obtained from the United States Department of Agriculture publication *Composition of Foods, Agricultural Handbook No. 8*.

FOOD CATEGORIES—
WHAT IS SAFE AND WHAT IS NOT

As in all food control programs, there are certain categories of food that lend themselves easily to positive or negative recognition. Foods that are called "safe" are those that will cause you no trouble. Foods that are "possible" should be considered seriously before you indulge in them. Read the labels on all cans and packages to see if the food is no-salt, low-sodium, or salt-free. As for those foods you should "stay away from," you should memorize them and never go near them.

Although the listing that follows is not complete, it can be used as a guideline to make your life easier.

SAFE FOODS

Beverages:
   Beer
   Cider
   Cordials
   Fruit juices
   Fruit nectars
   Liqueurs
   Spirits
   Wines
Condiments:
   Carob
   Herbs
   Spices

Dairy Products:
   Cream
   Yogurt
Fruits:
   All fresh fruits
Poultry:
   Chicken
   Duck
   Turkey
Vegetables:
   All fresh vegetables, unless mentioned in other lists

POSSIBLE FOODS

(Check with your doctor, use your common sense, and read the labels on the foods you purchase to determine if they are no-salt, low-sodium, or salt-free.)

Baked Goods:
Breads
Cakes and cake mixes
Cookies and cookie mixes
Pancakes
Rolls or muffins
Waffles

Beverages:
Buttermilk

Condiments:
Bouillon cubes
Catsup
Chili sauce
Horseradish
Mayonnaise
Meat tenderizer
Mustard
Pickles
Relish
Tomato paste

Dairy Products:
Butter
Cheese
Ice cream
Sherbet

Fish and Seafood:
Canned fish

Fruits:
Dried fruits
Canned fruits
Frozen fruits

Meat:
Beef
Lamb
Pork
Canned soups and stews

Vegetables:
Canned vegetables
Frozen vegetables

STAY-AWAY-FROM FOODS

Baked Goods:
Breads
Cakes and cake mixes
Cookies and cookie mixes
Crackers
Pancakes
Rolls and muffins
(packaged or frozen)
Snack foods
Waffles (frozen)

Beverages:
Carbonated drinks
Chocolate milk
Cocoa
Milk shakes

*Low-sodium variety only.

Condiments:
- A-1 Sauce
- Celery salt
- Chutney
- Cocoa powder
- Garlic salt
- Gelatins (flavored)
- Lemon pepper
- Meat extracts
- Molasses
- MSG
- Olives
- Onion salt
- Rennet tablets
- Salt
- Salted nuts
- Soy sauce
- Sugar substitutes
- Worcestershire sauce

Dairy Products:
- Butter
- Cheese
- Ice cream
- Sherbet

Fish and Seafood:
- Anchovies
- Canned fish
- Caviar
- Clams
- Cod (salt or dried)
- Crabs
- Frozen fish
- Herring
- Lobster
- Salted fish
- Sardines
- Scallops
- Shellfish
- Shrimp
- Smoked fish

Meat:
- Bacon
- Bologna
- Brains
- Chipped beef
- Frankfurters
- Ham
- Kidneys
- Kosher meats
- Liverwurst
- Pickled meats
- Salami
- Salted meats
- Salt pork
- Sausage
- Smoked meats
- Spiced meats

Vegetables:
- Artichokes
- Beets
- Canned vegetables (unless mentioned in other lists)
- Celery
- Kale
- Sauerkraut

11

HOW TO GIVE UP
SALT AND NOT TASTE

When you have to cut down or give up salt, there is no reason that your taste buds have to suffer. There are numerous ways to season your food without using salt. For instance, the use of wine as a salt substitute and for seasoning at the table and in the kitchen offers a never-ending number of flavoring possibilities. I put dry sherry in a shaker bottle and put it on the table as a substitute for salt. Take a used salad dressing bottle and wash it well. Fill with dry sherry and try it on eggs, vegetables and meats. A quick sprinkle will wake up your taste buds.

The use of herbs and spices as a substitute for salt also offers a rainbow of taste experiences. Here is an extensive list of the different herbs and spices and the foods in which they can be used.

ALLSPICE

Baked Goods: baked pudding; cakes; coffee cake; cookies; gingerbread; mince pies; pumpkin pie; sweet rolls. *Beverages*: cranberry juice; tomato juice. *Condiments*: catsup; chili sauce; ham glaze. *Dairy Products*: none. *Fish and Seafood*: poached fish. *Fruits*: fruit compote; fruit salad. *Meat*: ham patties; meatballs; meatloaf; pot-roasted beef, lamb, and veal; stewed beef, lamb, and veal. *Poultry*: braised chicken; chicken fricassee; chicken pie; roast duck; stewed duck; turkey fricassee; turkey pie. *Sauces*: dessert; meat; tomato. *Soups*: chicken; consomme; fish chowder; potato; turtle; vegetable. *Vegetables*: beets; cabbage salad; carrots; parsnips; spinach; sweet potatoes; turnips; winter squash.

ANISE

Baked Goods: apple pie; cakes; coffee cake; cookies; sweet rolls. *Beverages*: fruit juice. *Condiments*: none. *Dairy Products*: cheese canapes; cottage cheese; mild-flavored cheeses; whipped cream. *Fish and Seafood*: shellfish canapes. *Fruits*: baked apples; fruit compote; fruit salad; fruit soup. *Meat*: stewed beef and veal. *Poultry*: braised chicken; chicken pilaf; duck pilaf; roast duck. *Sauces*: dessert; French dressing. *Soups*: none. *Vegetables*: cabbage salad.

BASIL

Baked Goods: pizza; yeast breads. *Beverages*: tomato juice; vegetable juice. *Condiments*: none. *Dairy Products*: egg salad; scrambled eggs; stuffed eggs; Welsh rarebit. *Fish and Seafood*: crab cakes; seafood cocktail; seafood salad; shrimp salad; lobster salad; stewed fish and shellfish. *Fruits*: none. *Meat*: hamburgers; meatballs; meat pot pies; broiled lamb chops; roasted beef, lamb, and veal. *Poultry*: fried chicken. *Sauces*: butter; cheese; French dressing; spaghetti; tomato. *Soups*: green pea; minestrone; potato; spinach; split pea; turtle; vegetable. *Vegetables*: asparagus; aspic salad; beets; broccoli; cabbage; carrots; celery; cucumber; eggplant; peas; spinach; tomatoes; tomato salad; turnips; vegetable salad; winter squash.

BAY LEAF

Baked Goods: none. *Beverages*: tomato juice. *Condiments*: none. *Dairy Products*: none. *Fish and Seafood*: court bouillon; boiled lobster; pickled fish; poached fish; broiled shrimp. *Fruits*: none. *Meat*: braised tongue; pot-roasted beef, lamb, and veal; pot-roasted venison; stewed beef, lamb, and veal; stewed rabbit. *Poultry*: chicken fricassee; stewed chicken. *Sauces*: meat; spaghetti; tomato. *Soups*: bouillabaisse; chicken; consomme; vegetable. *Vegetables*: aspic salad; molded vegetable salad; vegetable salad.

CARAWAY SEED

Baked Goods: apple pie; cakes; coffee cake; cookies; onion bread; pumpernickel bread; rolls; rye bread; sweet rolls. *Beverages*: tomato juice. *Condiments*: canape spreads; sandwich spreads. *Dairy Products*: cheese omelets; cheese spreads; cottage cheese salad; plain omelets. *Fish and Seafood*: boiled crab; boiled lobster; broiled fish; poached fish; stuffed fish. *Fruits*: none. *Meat*: roast beef; roast pork; sauerbraten; stewed beef. *Poultry*: roast goose. *Sauces*: butter (for noodles, spaghetti, and vegetables); French dressing; sour cream dressing. *Soups*: cabbage; cucumber; potato. *Vegetables*: cabbage; carrots; celery; coleslaw; cucumbers; cucumber salad; onions; potatoes; tomatoes; tomato salad; turnips.

CARDAMOM SEED

Baked Goods: apple pie; cakes; coffee cake; cookies; Danish pastry; Lucia buns; pumpkin pie; sweet yeast breads. *Beverages*: none. *Condiments*: none. *Dairy Products*: none. *Fish and Seafood*: curried shrimp. *Fruits*: baked apples; fruit compote; melon salads (except watermelon). *Meat*: curried beef, lamb, pork, and veal. *Poultry*: curried chicken; stewed chicken. *Sauces*: hard; lemon; orange. *Soups*: none. *Vegetables*: carrots; pumpkin; sweet potatoes; winter squash.

CAYENNE

Baked Goods: cheese straws; cheese wafers. *Beverages*: none. *Condiments*: barbecue sauce. *Dairy Products*: cheese fondue; cheese soufflé; cheese spreads; cottage cheese salad; egg salad; macaroni and cheese; plain omelet; stuffed eggs; Welsh rarebit. *Fish and Seafood*: boiled crab; boiled lobster; boiled shrimp; broiled lobster; broiled shrimp; seafood salad. *Fruits*: none. *Meat*: beef and pork paprikash; curried beef, lamb, pork, and veal; ham croquettes; ham soufflé; pork sausage patties. *Poultry*: barbecued chicken; broiled chicken; curried chicken. *Sauces*: cheese; spaghetti; tomato. *Soups*: Brunswick stew; vegetable. *Vegetables*: cabbage; collard greens; guacamole; kale; kidney bean salad; turnip greens.

14

CELERY SEED

Baked Goods: cheese straws; cheese wafers. *Beverages*: clam juice cocktail; tomato juice. *Condiments*: none. *Dairy Products*: cheese soufflé; cheese spreads; scrambled eggs; plain omelet. *Fish and Seafood*: none. *Fruits*: none. *Meat*: meatloaf; pot-roasted beef, lamb, and veal; stewed beef, lamb, and veal. *Poultry*: chicken fricassee. *Sauces*: celery; French dressing; tomato. *Soups*: fish bisque; fish chowder; vegetable bisque. *Vegetables*: beets; braised lettuce; cabbage; coleslaw; cucumbers.

CHERVIL

Baked Goods: herb bread. *Beverages*: none. *Condiments*: none. *Dairy Products*: cottage cheese salad; cream cheese spread; egg salad; plain omelet; scrambled eggs; shirred eggs. *Fish and Seafood*: boiled lobster; boiled shrimp; broiled scallops; steamed clams. *Fruits*: none. *Meat*: none. *Poultry*: broiled chicken; chicken salad. *Sauces*: bearnaise; salad dressing; tomato; vinaigrette dressing. *Soups*: cream of potato; cream of spinach. *Vegetables*: beets; celery, cucumber salad; lettuce salad; potatoes; tomatoes; tomato salad; vegetable salad.

CHILI POWDER

Baked Goods: biscuits; French bread. *Beverages*: tomato juice. *Condiments*: cocktail sauce. *Dairy Products*: cheese dip; cheese fondue; cheese spreads; cottage cheese salad; egg salad; plain omelet; scrambled eggs; stuffed eggs; Welsh rarebit. *Fish and Seafood*: boiled lobster; boiled shrimp; broiled fish; seafood salad. *Fruits*: none. *Meat*: chili con carne; hamburgers; meatballs; meatloaf; stewed beef; tamale pie. *Poultry*: barbecued chicken; broiled chicken; chicken casseroles; fried chicken. *Sauces*: barbecue; cheese; salad dressing; spaghetti; tomato. *Soups*: bean puree; black bean; green pea; tomato. *Vegetables*: corn; eggplant; guacamole; lima beans; mixed vegetable salad; onions; potato salad; tomatoes.

CINNAMON

Baked Goods: apple pie; biscuits; cakes; chocolate cake; coffee cake; cookies; cranberry bread; gingerbread; pumpkin bread; pumpkin pie; rice pudding; sweet buns; sweet rolls; tea loaf. *Beverages*: cranberry juice; tomato juice. *Condiments*: cranberry sauce. *Dairy Products*: none. *Fish and Seafood*: none. *Fruits*: applesauce; baked apples; fruit compote; spiced jellied fruit salads; stewed apples. *Meat*: sauerbraten; stewed beef. *Poultry*: none. *Sauces*: chocolate; lemon; orange; raisin; spaghetti; tomato. *Soups*: fruit. *Vegetables*: beets; carrots; onions; pumpkin; sweet potatoes; tomatoes; winter squash.

CLOVES

Baked Goods: baked puddings; cakes; chocolate cake; coffee cake; cookies; gingerbread; sweet rolls; tea loaf; yeast bread. *Beverages*: cranberry juice; tomato juice. *Condiments*: catsup; chili sauce. *Dairy Products*: none. *Fish and Seafood*: none. *Fruits*: applesauce; fruit compote; spiced fruit salads; spiced jellied fruit salads. *Meat*: baked ham; boiled tongue; corned beef; meat stock; roast pork; stewed beef. *Poultry*: none. *Sauces*: chocolate; raisin; tomato. *Soups*: chicken; onion. *Vegetables*: beets; carrots; onions; pumpkin; sweet potatoes; winter squash.

CORIANDER

Baked Goods: apple pie; biscuits; cakes; cookies; gingerbread; sweet rolls. *Beverages*: none. *Condiments*: none. *Dairy Products*: curried eggs; egg salad; plain omelet; scrambled eggs. *Fish and Seafood*: none. *Fruits*: baked apples. *Meat*: curried beef, lamb, pork, and veal; meatballs; meat stock; pork sausage patties. *Poultry*: chicken stock; curried chicken; poultry stuffing. *Sauces*: salad dressing. *Soups*: split pea. *Vegetables*: cauliflower; mixed green salad; onions; spinach; tomatoes.

CUMIN SEED

Baked Goods: cakes; cookies. *Beverages*: none. *Condiments*: none. *Dairy Products*: cheese canapes; cheese spreads; curried eggs; egg canapes; stuffed eggs. *Fish and Seafood*: curried fish; curried seafood. *Fruits*: none. *Meat*: curried beef, lamb, pork, and veal; meatballs; meatloaf. *Poultry*: curried chicken; curried turkey; poultry stuffing. *Sauces*: curry; salad dressings (for fruit or chicken). *Soups*: none. *Vegetables*: none.

CURRY POWDER

Baked Goods: apple pie; French bread. *Beverages*: none. *Condiments*: none. *Dairy Products*: cheese fondue; cottage cheese salad; cream cheese spread; curried eggs; egg salad; macaroni and cheese; scrambled eggs; stuffed eggs. *Fish and Seafood*: boiled lobster; broiled fish; crab cakes; curried shrimp; seafood salad; seafood stuffing. *Fruits*: fruit compote; fruit salad. *Meat*: curried beef, lamb, pork, and veal; meatballs; meatloaf; roast lamb; roast pork; stewed lamb; stewed pork. *Poultry*: chicken salad; curried chicken; curried duck; poultry stuffing; roast chicken. *Sauces*: butter; celery; cheese; egg; onion; salad dressing. *Soups*: chicken; consomme; split pea; tomato; turtle; vegetable. *Vegetables*: beets; carrots; parsnips; sweet potatoes; turnips; winter squash.

DILL SEED

Baked Goods: dill bread; green apple pie; onion bread; onion rolls; yeast loaf. *Beverages*: tomato juice; vegetable juice. *Condiments*: none. *Dairy Products*: cottage cheese salad; cream cheese spread; egg salad; stuffed eggs. *Fish and Seafood*: broiled scallops; broiled shrimp; fish balls; fish loaf; seafood and rice casseroles. *Fruits*: none. *Meat*: broiled lamb chops; roast lamb; stewed lamb. *Poultry*: chicken and rice casseroles; creamed chicken. *Sauces*: butter; fish; French dressing; gravy; sour cream. *Soups*: fruit. *Vegetables*: cabbage salad; cucumber salad; potato salad; tomato salad; vegetable salad.

FENNEL SEED

Baked Goods: apple pie; cakes; cookies; muffins; yeast bread. *Beverages*: none. *Condiments*: none. *Dairy Products*: none. *Fish and Seafood*: baked fish; baked scallops; baked shrimp; poached fish; seafood pilaf; seafood salad. *Fruits*: baked apples; stewed apples. *Meat*: Italian sausage; stewed beef, lamb, and pork. *Poultry*: chicken pilaf; duck pilaf. *Sauces*: dessert; sauces for ham, pork, and tongue. *Soups*: cabbage; potato. *Vegetables*: cabbage; cucumbers; mixed green salad; onions; potatoes.

GINGER

Baked Goods: baked pudding; cakes; cookies; gingerbread; Indian pudding; pumpkin bread; sweet rolls; tea loaf. *Beverages*: apple juice; prune juice. *Condiments*: none. *Dairy Products*: macaroni and cheese. *Fish and Seafood*: none. *Fruits*: cantaloupe; stewed pears. *Meat*: oriental meat dishes; pot-roasted beef, lamb, and pork; roasted beef, lamb, and pork; stewed beef, lamb, and pork. *Poultry*: chicken casseroles; duck casseroles; fried chicken; roasted chicken; roasted duck. *Sauces*: dessert; French dressing; sauces for ham, pork, and tongue. *Soups*: none. *Vegetables*: carrots; sweet potatoes; winter squash.

ITALIAN SEASONING

Baked Goods: herb bread. *Beverages*: clam juice cocktail; tomato juice; vegetable juice. *Condiments*: none. *Dairy Products*: cheese omelet; cheese soufflé; macaroni and cheese; plain omelet; scrambled eggs. *Fish and Seafood*: baked fish; broiled fish; seafood salad; seafood stuffing. *Fruits*: none. *Meat*: broiled pork chops; fried pork chops; pot-roasted beef, lamb, and veal; stewed beef, lamb, and veal. *Poultry*: chicken fricassee; chicken pie; poultry stuffing; turkey pie. *Sauces*: cheese; French dressing; gravy; spaghetti; tomato. *Soups*: fish chowder; potato; vegetable. *Vegetables*: eggplant; tomatoes; vegetable salad; winter squash.

MACE

Baked Goods: banana bread; chocolate cake; cookies; doughnuts; pound cake; spice cake; sweet yeast rolls; tea loaf; yeast bread. *Beverages*: none. *Condiments*: none. *Dairy Products*: whipped cream. *Fish and Sea-*

food: none. *Fruits*: none. *Meat*: meatloaf; sautéed veal chops. *Poultry*: chicken fricassee. *Sauces*: dessert; sauces for chicken and fish. *Soups*: bean; clam bisque; oyster stew. *Vegetables*: broccoli; brussels sprouts; cabbage.

MARJORAM

Baked Goods: herb bread. *Beverages*: tomato juice. *Condiments*: none. *Dairy Products*: egg salad; plain omelet; scrambled eggs; sharp-cheese spreads. *Fish and Seafood*: baked fish; boiled shrimp; broiled fish; broiled shrimp; crab cakes; seafood salad; seafood stuffing. *Fruits*: none. *Meat*: liver and onions; meatloaf; pot-roasted beef and lamb; stewed beef and lamb. *Poultry*: chicken and duck liver pâté; chicken fricassee; chicken salad; chopped chicken liver; fried chicken; poultry stuffing; roast chicken; roast duck; roast turkey. *Sauces*: butter; French dressing; gravy; sauces for seafood; spaghetti; tomato. *Soups*: chicken; cream of celery; cream of chicken; cream of spinach; onion; potato. *Vegetables*: celery; collard greens; green peas; onions; potatoes; tomatoes; turnip greens.

MINT

Baked Goods: none. *Beverages*: fruit juice. *Condiments*: none. *Dairy Products*: cream cheese spread. *Fish and Seafood*: none. *Fruits*: fruit salad; melon ball salad. *Meat*: lamb stew. *Poultry*: none. *Sauces*: dessert; sauce for roast lamb. *Soups*: cream of pea. *Vegetables*: carrots; coleslaw; green peas.

MUSTARD

Baked Goods: cheese yeast bread; gingerbread; molasses cookies; spice cake. *Beverages*: none. *Condiments*: none. *Dairy Products*: egg salad; stuffed eggs. *Fish and Seafood*: shrimp cocktail. *Fruits*: none. *Meat*: ham; hamburgers; meatballs; meatloaf; meat salads; pork roast. *Poultry*: deviled chicken. *Sauces*: boiled salad dressing; cheese; egg; French dressing; gravy; vegetable. *Soups*: bisques; chowders. *Vegetables*: beets; braised lettuce; cabbage; cucumber.

NUTMEG

Baked Goods: apple pie; baked custard; baked pudding; banana bread; cakes; cookies; doughnuts; pumpkin pie; sweet breads; sweet rolls; tea loaf. *Beverages*: none. *Condiments*: none. *Dairy Products*: eggnog. *Fish and Seafood*: none. *Fruits*: applesauce; baked apples; fruit compote. *Meat*: beef pot pie; meatloaf; shepherd's pie. *Poultry*: deviled chicken. *Sauces*: hard. *Soups*: black bean; potato; split pea; tomato. *Vegetables*: corn; eggplant; onions; string beans; tomatoes.

OREGANO

Baked Goods: herb bread; pizza. *Beverages*: tomato juice; vegetable juice. *Condiments*: none. *Dairy Products*: cheese spreads; egg salad; plain omelet; stuffed eggs. *Fish and Seafood*: broiled fish; broiled seafood; seafood stuffing; shrimp salad. *Fruits*: none. *Meat*: chili con carne; hamburgers; meat salads; roasted beef, lamb, and pork; stewed beef, lamb, and pork. *Poultry*: roast Guinea hen; roast pheasant. *Sauces*: butter; salad dressing; sauce for shrimp; spaghetti; tomato. *Soups*: bean; lentil; tomato; vegetable. *Vegetables*: broccoli; cabbage; eggplant; guacamole; kidney bean salad; tomatoes; tomato salad; vegetable salad.

PAPRIKA

Baked Goods: none. *Beverages*: none. *Condiments*: none. *Dairy Products*: garnish for salads and spreads. *Fish and Seafood*: garnish for baked or broiled fish and seafood. *Fruits*: none. *Meat*: beef, pork, and veal paprikash. *Poultry*: chicken paprikash. *Sauces*: barbecue; butter; cucumber; salad dressing. *Soups*: split pea. *Vegetables*: cauliflower; corn; onions; potatoes; spinach.

PARSLEY

Baked Goods: biscuits; herb bread. *Beverages*: clam juice cocktail; tomato juice. *Condiments*: tartar sauce. *Dairy Products*: cheese dip; cheese soufflé; cottage cheese salad; cream cheese spread; creamed eggs; egg salad; plain omelet; scrambled eggs; stuffed eggs. *Fish and Seafood*: court bouillon; fish stew; lobster Thermidor; paella; seafood salad; seafood stew; seafood stuffing. *Fruits*: none. *Meat*: meatloaf; meat pot pies; meat stock; stewed beef, lamb, and veal. *Poultry*: chicken fricassee; chicken pot pie; chicken stock; poultry stuffing; turkey pot pie. *Sauces*: butter; bordelaise; remoulade; spaghetti; tomato. *Soups*: beef; chicken; green pea; lentil; split pea; vegetable. *Vegetables*: aspic salad; beets; cabbage; carrots; cauliflower; celery; eggplant; onions; potatoes; potato salad; turnips; vegetable salads.

PEPPER, BLACK

Baked Goods: crackling bread; Easter bread; gingerbread; Italian yeast bread; spice cake; spice cookies; spice tea loaf. *Beverages*: tomato juice; vegetable juice. *Condiments*: none. *Dairy Products*: cheese soufflé; cheese spreads; cottage cheese salad; creamed eggs; egg salad; plain omelet; scrambled eggs; stuffed eggs; Welsh rarebit. *Fish and Seafood*: baked fish; boiled lobster; boiled shrimp; broiled fish; crab cakes; fish salad; seafood salad. *Fruits*: none. *Meat*: meat salads; pâtés; pot-roasted beef, lamb, pork, and veal; roasted beef, lamb, pork, and veal; stewed beef, lamb, pork, and veal. *Poultry*: broiled chicken; chicken fricassee; chicken salad; fried chicken; roast chicken; roast duck; roast turkey. *Sauces*: barbecue; butter; cheese; cream; egg; spaghetti; tomato. *Soups*: bisques; chowders; fruit; vegetable. *Vegetables*: beets; carrots; onions; potatoes; rutabagas; sweet potatoes; tomatoes; winter squash.

PEPPER, WHITE

Baked Goods: crackling bread; Easter bread; gingerbread; Italian yeast bread; spice cake; spice cookies; spice tea loaf. *Beverages*: tomato juice; vegetable juice. *Condiments*: none. *Dairy Products*: cheese soufflé; cheese spreads; cottage cheese salad; creamed eggs; egg salad; plain omelet; scrambled eggs. *Fish and Seafood*: baked fish; boiled lobster; boiled shrimp; broiled fish; crab cakes; fish salad; seafood salad. *Fruits*: none. *Meat*: meat salads; pâtés; pot-roasted beef, lamb, pork, and veal; roasted beef, lamb, pork, and veal; stewed beef, lamb, pork, and veal; veal stock. *Poultry*: broiled chicken; chicken fricassee; chicken salad; chicken stock; fried chicken; roast chicken; roast duck; roast turkey. *Sauces*: barbecue; butter; cheese; cream; egg; spaghetti; tomato. *Soups*: bisques; chowders; vegetable. *Vegetables*: beets; carrots; onions; potatoes; sweet potatoes; tomatoes; winter squash.

POULTRY SEASONING

Baked Goods: biscuits. *Beverages*: none. *Condiments*: none. *Dairy Products*: egg salad. *Fish and Seafood*: none. *Fruits*: none. *Meat*: casseroles; meat croquettes; stews. *Poultry*: chicken croquettes; chicken fricassee; chicken salad; poultry stuffing; roast chicken; roast duck; roast turkey; turkey croquettes; turkey salad. *Sauces*: chicken and turkey gravy; cream. *Soups*: bisques; chicken; chowders. *Vegetables*: cauliflower; potatoes; turnips.

ROSEMARY

Baked Goods: yeast loaf. *Beverages*: none. *Condiments*: none. *Dairy Products*: plain omelet; scrambled eggs; shirred eggs; soufflé. *Fish and Seafood*: broiled fish; broiled scallops; fish croquettes; seafood salad; tuna loaf. *Fruits*: fruit salad. *Meat*: none. *Poultry*: chicken salad; roast chicken; turkey salad. *Sauces*: butter; cream; French dressing. *Soups*: chicken; chowders; lamb and bean; tomato. *Vegetables*: cauliflower; potatoes; turnips.

SAFFRON

Baked Goods: tea loaf; yeast bread; yeast rolls. *Beverages*: none. *Condiments*: none. *Dairy Products*: cream cheese spread; creamed eggs; scrambled eggs. *Fish and Seafood*: paella; seafood and rice casseroles; shrimp pilaf. *Fruits*: none. *Meat*: none. *Poultry*: arroz con pollo; chicken pilaf; roast chicken; roast duck; turkey pilaf. *Sauces*: tomato. *Soups*: none. *Vegetables*: none.

SAGE

Baked Goods: biscuits; corn bread. *Beverages*: clam juice cocktail; tomato juice. *Condiments*: none. *Dairy Products*: cheese fondue; cheese omelet. *Fish and Seafood*: baked fish. *Fruits*: none. *Meat*: sausage patties; stewed pork and veal. *Poultry*: chicken salad; poultry stuffing; roast chicken; roast turkey; turkey salad. *Sauces*: butter sauce for fish; chicken and turkey gravy; cream sauce for poultry; salad dressing. *Soups*: chicken; chowders; turkey. *Vegetables*: beets; celery; onions; summer squash; tomatoes; winter squash.

SAVORY

Baked Goods: none. *Beverages*: tomato juice; vegetable juice. *Condiments*: none. *Dairy Products*: plain omelet; scrambled eggs; stuffed eggs. *Fish and Seafood*: broiled fish. *Fruits*: none. *Meat*: hamburgers; meat pot pies; meat stock; roasted beef, lamb, pork, and veal. *Poultry*: broiled chicken; roast chicken; roast turkey. *Sauces*: butter sauces for fish and poultry; cream sauces for fish and poultry; salad dressing. *Soups*: bean; chicken; cucumber; potato; tomato. *Vegetables*: carrots; cucumbers; potatoes; string beans; tomatoes.

SESAME SEED

Baked Goods: cakes; coffee cake; cookies; quick breads; sweet rolls; tea loaf; yeast rolls. *Beverages*: none. *Condiments*: none. *Dairy Products*: cheese omelet, cheese spreads; scrambled eggs. *Fish and Seafood*: baked fish; broiled fish; broiled lobster; broiled shrimp; crab salad. *Fruits*: fruit salad. *Meat*: none. *Poultry*: chicken salad; roast chicken; roast duck. *Sauces*: butter; salad dressing. *Soups*: none. *Vegetables*: corn; summer squash; tomato salad; winter squash.

TARRAGON

Baked Goods: none. *Beverages*: tomato juice; vegetable juice. *Condiments*: none. *Dairy Products*: creamed eggs; egg salad; plain omelet; scrambled eggs. *Fish and Seafood*: broiled fish; broiled shrimp. *Fruits*: none. *Meat*: pot-roasted lamb and veal; stewed lamb and veal. *Poultry*: chicken liver pâté; chicken fricassee; chicken salad; roast chicken; stewed chicken. *Sauces*: cream sauce for chicken, fish, and seafood. *Soups*: chicken; mushroom; split pea; tomato. *Vegetables*: beets; carrots; mixed green salad; onions; potato salad; string beans; summer squash; tomatoes; tomato salad; winter squash.

THYME

Baked Goods: biscuits; corn bread; yeast bread. *Beverages*: fruit juice; tomato juice. *Condiments*: none. *Dairy Products*: cottage cheese salad; egg salad; scrambled eggs; stuffed eggs. *Fish and Seafood*: broiled fish; broiled lobster; broiled scallops; broiled shrimp; crab cakes; tuna salad. *Fruits*: none. *Meat*: ham salad; meatballs; meat croquettes; meatloaf; pot-roasted beef, lamb, pork, and veal; roasted beef, lamb, pork, and veal; stewed beef, lamb, pork, and veal. *Poultry*: chicken fricassee; chicken salad; fried chicken; roast chicken; roast duck. *Sauces*: cream sauce for poultry and seafood; creole; gravy. *Soups*: bisques; chicken; chowders; mushroom; tomato; vegetable. *Vegetables*: aspic salad; beets; beet salad; carrots; onions; string beans; summer squash; tomato salad; winter squash.

TUMERIC

Baked Goods: none. *Beverages*: none. *Condiments*: none. *Dairy Products*: creamed eggs; egg salad; stuffed eggs. *Fish and Seafood*: baked fish; fish and rice casseroles; shrimp pilaf. *Fruits*: none. *Meat*: curried beef, lamb, and pork. *Poultry*: chicken pilaf; curried chicken; curried turkey; duck pilaf. *Sauces*: cream sauce for eggs, fish, seafood, and chicken. *Soups*: none. *Vegetables*: none.

HOW TO USE
THE SODIUM COUNTER

The following tables indicate in milligrams the amount of salt or potassium in 3.5 ounces or 100 grams of food.

For example: 1 raw apple weighing 3.5 ounces contains 1 mg of sodium and 10 mg of potassium

1 3.5-ounce serving of Apple brown betty contains 153 mg of sodium and 100 mg of potassium

Measures
1 pound = 16 ounces (oz)
1 ounce = 28.4 grams (g)
3.52 ounces = 100 grams (g)
1 gram = 1,000 milligrams (mg)

Note: "NA" in the listings denotes lack of reliable data for the amount of sodium or potassium believed to be present in measurable amounts. The numbers in parentheses denote computed values, usually from another form of the food or from a similar food.

SODIUM AND POTASSIUM COUNT
(in milligrams)

	SODIUM (MG PER 3.5 OZ OR 100 G)	POTASSIUM (MG PER 3.5 OZ OR 100 G)
Apples:		
Raw	1	10
Dehydrated, sulfured		
uncooked	7	730
Dried, sulfured		
Uncooked	5	569
Cooked:		
without added sugar	1	162
with added sugar	1	144
Apple brown betty	153	100
Apple butter	2	252
Apple juice, canned or bottled	1	101
Applesauce, canned:		
unsweetened or artificially sweetened	2	78
sweetened	2	65
Apricots:		
Raw	1	281
Candied	NA	NA
Canned, solids and liquid:		
Water pack, with or without artificial sweetener	1	246
Juice pack	1	362
Syrup pack:		
Light	1	239
Heavy	1	234
Dehydrated, sulfured:		
uncooked	33	1,260
cooked, fruit and liquid, sugar added	8	299
Dried, sulfured:		
uncooked	26	979
Apricot nectar, canned	Trace	151
Artichokes, globe or French:		
Cooked, boiled, drained	30	301
Asparagus:		
Cooked spears, boiled, drained	1	183
Canned spears:		
Green:		
Regular pack:		
Solids and liquid	236	166

26

	SODIUM (MG PER 3.5 OZ OR 100 G)	POTASSIUM (MG PER 3.5 OZ OR 100 G)
Asparagus continued		
Drained solids	236	166
Special dietary pack (low-sodium):		
Solids and liquid	3	166
Drained solids	3	166
Drained liquid	3	166
Frozen:		
Cuts and tips:		
Cooked, boiled and drained	1	220
Spears:		
Cooked, boiled and drained	1	238
Avocados, raw	4	604
Baby foods, strained or chopped:		
Cereals, precooked, dry, and other cereal products:		
Barley, added nutrients	452	413
High protein, added nutrients	653	1,078
Mixed, added nutrients	470	345
Oatmeal, added nutrients	437	374
Rice, added nutrients	530	208
Desserts, canned:		
Custard pudding, all flavors	150	94
Fruit pudding with starch base, milk &/or egg (banana, orange, or pineapple)	128	75
Dinners, canned:		
Cereal, vegetable, meat mixtures:		
Beef noodle dinner	269	159
Cereal, egg yolk & bacon	301	36
Chicken noodle dinner	297	42
Macaroni, tomatoes, meat & cereal	381	77
Split peas, vegetables, & ham or bacon	295	112
Vegetables & bacon, with cereal	282	130
Vegetables & beef, with cereal	307	143
Vegetables & chicken, with cereal	307	55
Vegetables & ham, with cereal	360	90

27

	SODIUM (MG PER 3.5 OZ OR 100 G)	POTASSIUM (MG PER 3.5. OZ OR 100 G)
Baby foods continued		
Vegetables & lamb, with cereal	269	148
Vegetables & liver, with cereal	236	162
Vegetables & liver, with bacon & cereal	284	131
Vegetables & turkey, with cereal	307	46
Meat or poultry:		
Beef with vegetables	304	113
Chicken with vegetables	265	71
Turkey with vegetables	348	122
Veal with vegetables	323	95
Fruits & fruit products, with or without thickening, canned:		
Applesauce	6	64
Applesauce & apricots	3–45*	105
Bananas (with tapioca or cornstarch, added ascorbic acid), strained	29	118
Bananas & pineapple (with tapioca or cornstarch)	59	72
Fruit dessert with tapioca (apricot, pineapple, &/or orange)	53	73
Peaches	4–75*	80
Pears	4	62
Pears & pineapple	4–75*	72
Plums with tapioca, strained	38	44
Prunes with tapioca	33	120
Meats, poultry, & eggs, canned:		
Beef:		
Strained	228	183
Junior	283	242
Beef heart	208	NA
Chicken	263	96
Egg yolks, strained	273	59
Egg yolks with ham or bacon	313	82
Lamb:		
Strained	241	181
Junior	294	228
Liver, strained	253	202
Liver and bacon, strained	302	192

*Depends on processing.

Baby foods continued	SODIUM (MG PER 3.5 OZ OR 100 G)	POTASSIUM (MG PER 3.5 OZ OR 100 G)
Pork:		
Strained	223	178
Junior	237	210
Veal:		
Strained	226	214
Junior	276	206
Vegetables, canned:		
Beans, green	213	93
Beets, strained	212	228
Carrots	169	181
Mixed vegetables, including vegetable soup	272	170
Peas, strained	194	100
Spinach, creamed	272	142
Squash	292	138
Sweet potatoes	187	180
Tomato soup, strained	294	300
Bacon, cured:		
Cooked, broiled or fried, drained	1,021	236
Canned	NA	NA
Bacon, Canadian:		
Cooked, broiled or fried, drained	2,555	482
Baking powders:		
Home use (list of ingredients on label indicates type of baking powder):		
Sodium aluminum sulfate:		
With monocalcium phosphate monohydrate	10,953	150
With monocalcium phosphate monohydrate & calcium carbonate	11,618	NA
With monocalcium phosphate monohydrate & calcium sulfate	10,000	NA
Straight phosphate	8,220	170
Tartrate:		
Cream of tartar, with tartaric acid	7,300	3,800
Special low-sodium preparation:		
Commercial powder	6*	10,948

*Value based on a single brand.

29

	SODIUM (MG PER 3.5 OZ OR 100 G)	POTASSIUM (MG PER 3.5 OZ OR 100 G)
Bamboo shoots, raw	NA	533
Bananas, common raw	1	370
Barbecue sauce	815	174
Barley, pearled:		
Light	3	60
Pot or Scotch	NA	296
Bass, black sea:		
Raw	68	256
Bass, striped:		
Raw	NA	NA
Beans, common, mature seeds, dry:		
White:		
Cooked (unsalted)	7	416
Canned, solids & liquid:		
With pork & tomato sauce	463	210
With pork & sweet sauce	380	NA
Without pork	338	268
Red:		
Cooked (unsalted)	3	340
Canned, solids & liquid	3	264
Beans, lima:		
Immature seeds:		
Cooked, boiled, drained	1	422
Canned:		
Regular pack:		
Solids & liquid	236*	222
Drained solids	236*	222
Special dietary pack (low-sodium):		
Solids & liquid	4	222
Drained solids	4	222
Frozen:		
Thick-seeded types, commonly called Fordhooks:		
Cooked, boiled, drained	101	426
Thin-seeded types, commonly called baby limas:		
Cooked, boiled, drained	129	394

*Estimated average based on the addition of salt in the amount of 0.6 percent of the finished product.

	SODIUM (MG PER 3.5 OZ OR 100 G)	POTASSIUM (MG PER 3.5 OZ OR 100 G)
Beans continued		
Mature seeds, dry:		
Cooked	2	612
Beans, mung:		
Mature seeds, dry, raw	6	1,028
Sprouted seeds:		
Uncooked	5	223
Cooked, boiled, drained	4	156
Beans, snap:		
Green:		
Raw	7	243
Cooked, boiled, drained	4	151
Canned:		
Regular pack:		
Solids & liquid	236*	95
Drained solids	236*	95
Specialty dietary·pack (low-sodium):		
Solids & liquid	2	95
Drained solids	2	95
Frozen:		
Cut, cooked, boiled, drained	1	152
French style, cooked, boiled, drained	2	136
Yellow or wax:		
Cooked, boiled, drained	3	151
Canned:		
Regular pack:		
Solids & liquid	236*	95
Drained solids	236*	95
Special dietary pack (low-sodium):		
Solids & liquid	2	95
Drained solids	2	95
Frozen, cut:		
Cooked, boiled, drained	4	151
Beans & frankfurters, canned	539	262
Beef:		
Retail cuts, trimmed to retail level:		

*Estimated average based on the addition of salt in the amount of 0.6 percent of the finished product.

	SODIUM (MG PER 3.5 OZ OR 100 G)	POTASSIUM (MG PER 3.5 OZ OR 100 G)
Beef continued		
Chuck cuts:		
Entire chuck, 1st–5th ribs, arm & neck:		
Choice grade:		
Total edible:		
Cooked, braised, or pot-roasted	60	370
Chuck rib, 5th:		
Choice grade:		
Total edible:		
Cooked, braised	60	370
Good grade:		
Total edible:		
Cooked, braised	60	370
Arm:		
Choice grade:		
Total edible:		
Cooked, braised, or pot-roasted	60	370
Good grade:		
Total edible:		
Cooked, braised, or pot-roasted	60	370
Flank steak:		
Choice grade:		
Total edible:		
Cooked, braised	60	370
Good grade:		
Total edible:		
Cooked, braised	60	370
Hindshank:		
Choice grade:		
Total edible:		
Cooked, simmered	60	370
Good grade:		
Total edible:		
Cooked, simmered	60	370
Loin or short loin:		
Porterhouse steak:		
Choice grade:		
Total edible:		
Cooked, broiled	60	370

	SODIUM (MG PER 3.5 OZ OR 100 G)	POTASSIUM (MG PER 3.5 OZ OR 100 G)
Beef continued		
Good grade:		
Total edible:		
Cooked, broiled	60	370
T-bone steak:		
Choice grade:		
Total edible:		
Cooked, broiled	60	370
Good grade:		
Total edible:		
Cooked, broiled	60	370
Club steak:		
Choice grade:		
Total edible:		
Cooked, broiled	60	370
Good grade:		
Total edible:		
Cooked, broiled	60	370
Loin end or sirloin:		
Wedge & round-bone sirloin steak:		
Choice grade:		
Total edible:		
Cooked, broiled	60	370
Good grade:		
Total edible:		
Cooked, broiled	60	370
Double-bone sirloin steak:		
Choice grade:		
Total edible:		
Cooked, broiled	60	370
Good grade:		
Total edible:		
Cooked, broiled	60	370
Hipbone sirloin steak:		
Choice grade:		
Total edible:		
Cooked, broiled	60	370
Good grade:		
Total edible:		
Cooked, broiled	60	370
Short plate:		
Choice grade:		
Total edible:		
Cooked, simmered	60	370

	SODIUM (MG PER 3.5 OZ OR 100 G)	POTASSIUM (MG PER 3.5 OZ OR 100 G)
Beef continued		
Good grade:		
Total edible:		
Cooked, simmered	60	370
Rib:		
Entire rib, 6th–12th ribs:		
Choice grade:		
Total edible:		
Cooked, roasted	60	370
Ribs, 11th–12th:		
Choice grade:		
Total edible:		
Cooked, roasted	60	370
Good grade:		
Total edible:		
Cooked, roasted	60	370
Rib, 6th or blade:		
Choice grade:		
Total edible:		
Cooked, braised	60	370
Good grade:		
Total edible:		
Cooked, braised	60	370
Round, entire (round & heel of round):		
Choice grade:		
Total edible:		
Cooked, broiled	60	370
Rump:		
Choice grade:		
Total edible:		
Cooked, roasted	60	370
Good grade:		
Total edible:		
Cooked, roasted	60	370
Hamburger (ground beef):		
Lean:		
Cooked	48	558
Regular ground:		
Cooked	47	450
Beef & vegetable stew:		
Cooked (home recipe, with lean beef chuck)	37	250
Beef, canned, roast beef	NA	259

	SODIUM (MG PER 3.5 OZ OR 100 G)	POTASSIUM (MG PER 3.5 OZ OR 100 G)
Beef, corned, boneless:		
Cooked, medium-fat	1,740	150
Canned:		
Fat	NA	NA
Medium-fat	NA	NA
Lean	NA	NA
Canned corned-beef hash (with potato)	540	200
Beef, dried, chipped:		
Cooked, creamed	716	153
Beef pot pie:		
Home-prepared, baked	284	159
Commercial, frozen, unheated	366	93
Beets, common, red:		
Cooked, boiled, drained	43	208
Canned:		
Regular pack:		
Solids & liquid	236*	167
Drained solids	236*	167
Special dietary pack (low-sodium)		
Solids & liquid	46	167
Drained solids	46	167
Beet greens, common:		
Raw	130	570
Cooked, boiled, drained	76	332
Beverages, alcoholic & carbonated nonalcoholic		
Alcoholic:		
Beer, alcohol 4.5% by volume	7	25
Gin, rum, vodka, whiskey:		
80-proof	1	2
86-proof	1	2
90-proof	1	2
94-proof	1	2
100-proof	1	2
Wines:		
Dessert, alcohol 18.8% by volume	4	75
Table, alcohol 12.2% by volume	5	92

*Estimated average based on the addition of salt in the amount of 0.6 percent of the finished product.

	SODIUM (MG PER 3.5 OZ OR 100 G)	POTASSIUM (MG PER 3.5 OZ OR 100 G)
Beverages continued		
Carbonated, nonalcoholic:		
Carbonated waters:		
Sweetened (quinine sodas)	NA	NA
Unsweetened (club sodas)	NA	NA
Cola type	NA	NA
Cream sodas	NA	NA
Fruit-flavored sodas (citrus, cherry, grape, strawberry, Tom Collins mixer, other)	NA	NA
Ginger ale, pale dry & golden	NA	NA
Root beer	NA	NA
Special dietary drinks with artificial sweetener (less than 1 calorie per ounce)	NA	NA
Biscuits, baking powder, baked from home recipe, made with:		
Enriched flour	626	117
Unenriched flour	626	117
Self-rising flour, enriched	660	64
Biscuit dough, commercial, with enriched flour:		
Chilled in cans	868	65
Frozen	910	86
Biscuit mix, with enriched flour & biscuits baked from mix:		
Mix, dry form	1,300	80
Biscuits, made with milk	973	116
Blackberries, including dewberries, boysenberries, and youngberries, raw	1	170
Blackberries, canned, solids & liquid:		
Water pack, with or without artificial sweetener	1	115
Juice pack	1	170
Syrup pack	1	110
Blackberry juice, canned, unsweetened	(1)	(170)
Blueberries:		
Raw	1	81
Canned, solids & liquid:		
Water pack, with or without artificial sweetener	1	60

	SODIUM (MG PER 3.5 OZ OR 100 G)	POTASSIUM (MG PER 3.5 OZ OR 100 G)
Blueberries continued		
Syrup pack, extra heavy	1	55
Frozen, not thawed		
Unsweetened	1	81
Sweetened	1	66
Bluefish:		
Raw:	74	NA
Cooked:		
Baked or broiled (prepared with butter or margarine)	104	NA
Fried (prepared with egg, milk, or water, & breadcrumbs)	126	NA
Bonito, including Atlantic, Pacific & striped, raw	NA	NA
Boston brown bread	251	292
Bouillon cubes or powder	24,000	100
Boysenberries:		
Canned, water pack, solids & liquid, with or without artificial sweetener	1	85
Frozen, not thawed:		
Unsweetened	1	153
Sweetened	1	105
Brains, all kinds (beef, calf, hog, sheep), raw	125	219
Bran:		
Added sugar & malt extract	1,060	1,070
Added sugar & defatted wheat germ	490	NA
Bran flakes (40% bran), added thiamine	925	NA
Bran flakes with raisins, added thiamine	800	NA
Brazil nuts	1	715
Breads:		
Cracked wheat	529	134
French or Vienna:		
Enriched	580	90
Unenriched	580	90
Italian:		
Enriched	585	74
Unenriched	585	74
Raisin	365	233

	SODIUM (MG PER 3.5 OZ OR 100 G)	POTASSIUM (MG PER 3.5 OZ OR 100 G)
Breads continued		
Rye:		
American (⅓ rye, ⅔ clear flour)	557	145
Pumpernickel	569	454
Salt-rising	265	67
White:		
Enriched, made with		
1%–2% nonfat dry milk	507	85
3%–4% nonfat dry milk*	507	105
5%–6% nonfat dry milk	495	121
Unenriched, made with		
1%–2% nonfat dry milk	507	85
3%–4% nonfat dry milk*	507	105
5%–6% nonfat dry milk	495	121
Whole wheat, made with		
2% nonfat dry milk	527	273
Water	530	256
Breadcrumbs, dry, grated	736	152
Bread pudding with raisins	201	215
Bread sticks (Vienna). See Salt sticks.		
Bread stuffing mix & stuffings prepared from mix:		
Mix, dry form	1,331	172
Stuffing:		
Dry, crumbly (prepared with water, table fat)	896	90
Moist (prepared with water, egg, table fat)	504	58
Breakfast cereals. See Corn, Oats, Rice, Wheat, Bran, Farina.		
Broadbeans, raw:		
Immature seeds	4	471
Mature seeds, dry	NA	NA
Broccoli:		
Raw spears	15	382
Cooked spears, boiled, drained	10	267
Frozen:		
Chopped:		
Cooked, boiled, drained	15	212

*When amount of nonfat dry milk in commercial bread is unknown, the values for bread with 3 to 4 percent nonfat dry milk are suggested.

	SODIUM (MG PER 3.5 OZ OR 100 G)	POTASSIUM (MG PER 3.5 OZ OR 100 G)
Broccoli continued		
Spears:		
Cooked, boiled, drained	12	220
Brussels sprouts:		
Cooked, boiled, drained	10	273
Frozen:		
Cooked, boiled, drained	14	295
Buckwheat:		
Whole grain	NA	448
Flour:		
Dark	NA	NA
Light	NA	320
Bulgur (parboiled wheat):		
Dry, commercial, made from		
Club wheat	NA	262
Hard red winter wheat	NA	229
White wheat	NA	310
Canned, made from hard red winter wheat:		
Unseasoned (processed, partially debranned, whole-kernel wheat with salt added)	599	87
Seasoned (processed, partially debranned, whole-kernel wheat with chicken fat, chicken stock base, dehydrated onion flakes, salt, monosodium glutamate, & herbs)	460	112
Butter:		
Salted	987	23
Unsalted	10	10
Buttermilk:		
Fluid, cultured (made from skim milk)	130	140
Cabbage, common varieties (Danish, domestic, & pointed types):		
Raw	20	233
Cooked, boiled until tender, drained:		
Shredded, cooked in small amount of water	14	163

	SODIUM (MG PER 3.5 OZ OR 100 G)	POTASSIUM (MG PER 3.5 OZ OR 100 G)
Cabbage continued		
Wedges, cooked in large amount of water	13	151
Red, raw	26	268
Savoy, raw	22	269
Cabbage, Chinese (also called celery cabbage or petsai), compact heading type, raw	23	253
Cabbage, spoon (also called white mustard cabbage or pakchoy), nonheading green leaf-type:		
Raw	26	306
Cooked, boiled, drained	18	214
Cakes:		
Baked from home recipes (unenriched cake flour unless otherwise specified):		
Angelfood	283	88
Boston cream pie	186	89
Caramel:		
Without icing	305	68
With caramel icing	252	64
Chocolate (devil's food):		
Without icing	294	140
With chocolate icing	235	154
With uncooked white icing	234	110
Cottage pudding, made with enriched flour:		
Without sauce	299	88
With chocolate sauce	233	140
With fruit sauce (strawberry)	233	93
Fruitcake, made with enriched flour:		
Dark	158	496
Light	193	233
Gingerbread, made with enriched flour	237	454
Plain cake or cupcake:		
Without icing	300	79
With chocolate icing	229	114
With boiled white icing	262	64
With uncooked white icing	227	61
Pound:		
Old-fashioned (equal		

	SODIUM (MG PER 3.5 OZ OR 100 G)	POTASSIUM (MG PER 3.5 OZ OR 100 G)
Cakes continued		
weights flour, sugar, table fat, eggs)	110	60
Modified	178	78
Sponge	167	87
White:		
Without icing	323	76
With coconut icing	257	106
With uncooked white icing	234	58
Yellow:		
Without icing	258	78
With caramel icing	226	73
With chocolate icing	208	108
Frozen, commercial, devil's food:		
With chocolate icing	420	119
With whipped-cream filling, chocolate icing	190	113
Cake mixes & cakes baked from mixes:		
Angelfood:		
Cake, made with water, flavorings	146	60
Chocolate malt:		
Cake, made with eggs, water, uncooked white icing	318	80
Coffee cake, with enriched flour:		
Cake, made with egg, milk	431	100
Cupcake:		
Cake, made with eggs, milk, without icing	453	84
Cake, made with eggs, milk, chocolate icing	335	117
Devil's food:		
Cake, made with eggs, water, chocolate icing	262	130
Gingerbread:		
Cake, made with water	304	274
Honey spice:		
Cake, made with eggs, water, caramel icing	245	88

	SODIUM (MG PER 3.5 OZ OR 100 G)	POTASSIUM (MG PER 3.5 OZ OR 100 G)
Cakes continued		
Marble:		
Cake, made with eggs, water, boiled white icing	259	122
White:		
Cake, made with egg whites, water, chocolate icing	227	116
Yellow:		
Cake, made with eggs, water, chocolate icing	227	109
Cake icings:		
Caramel	83	52
Chocolate	61	195
Coconut	118	167
White:		
Uncooked	49	18
Boiled	143	18
Cake icing mixes & icings made from mixes:		
Chocolate fudge:		
Icing, made with water, table fat	156	65
Creamy fudge (contains nonfat dry milk):		
Icing:		
Made with water	232	97
Made with water, table fat	321	89
Candied Fruits. See Apricots, Cherries, Citron, Figs, Gingerroot, Grapefruit peel, Lemon peel, Orange peel, Pear, and Pineapple.		
Candy:		
Butterscotch	66	2
Caramels:		
Plain or chocolate	226	192
Plain or chocolate, with nuts	203	233
Chocolate-flavored roll	197	123
Chocolate:		
Bittersweet	3	615
Semisweet	2	325
Sweet	33	269

	SODIUM (MG PER 3.5 OZ OR 100 G)	POTASSIUM (MG PER 3.5 OZ OR 100 G)
Candy continued		
Chocolate, milk:		
Plain	94	384
With almonds	80	442
With peanuts	66	487
Chocolate-coated:		
Almonds	59	546
Chocolate fudge	228	193
Chocolate fudge, with nuts	205	219
Coconut center	197	165
Fondant	185	91
Fudge, caramel & peanuts	204	301
Fudge, peanuts & caramel	128	222
Honeycombed hard candy, with peanut butter	163	225
Nougat & caramel	173	211
Peanuts	60	504
Raisins	64	603
Vanilla creams	182	178
Fondant	212	5
Fudge:		
Chocolate	190	147
Chocolate, with nuts	171	177
Vanilla	208	127
Vanilla, with nuts	187	114
Gum drops, starch jelly pieces	33	5
Hard	32	4
Jelly beans	12	1
Marshmallows	39	6
Mints, uncoated. See Fondant.	10	448
Peanut bars	10	448
Peanut brittle (no added salt or soda)	31	151
Sugar-coated:		
Almonds	20	255
Chocolate discs	72	250
Carob flour (St. Johnsbread)	NA	NA
Carrots:		
Raw	47	341
Cooked, boiled, drained	33	222
Canned:		
Regular pack:		
Solids & liquid	236*	120

*Estimated average based on the addition of salt in the amount of 0.6 percent of the finished product.

	SODIUM (MG PER 3.5 OZ OR 100 G)	POTASSIUM (MG PER 3.5 OZ OR 100 G)
Carrots continued		
Drained solids	236*	120
Special dietary pack (low-sodium):		
Solids & liquid	39	120
Drained solids	39	120
Cashew nuts		
Salted	200	464
Unsalted	15	464
Catfish, fresh water, raw	60	330
Cauliflower:		
Raw	13	295
Cooked, boiled, drained	9	206
Frozen:		
Cooked, boiled, drained	10	207
Caviar, sturgeon:		
Granular	2,200	180
Pressed	NA	NA
Celery, all, including green & yellow varieties:		
Raw	126	341
Cooked, boiled, drained	38	239
Chard, Swiss:		
Raw	147	550
Cooked, boiled, drained	86	321
Charlotte russe, with ladyfingers, whipped-cream filling	43	64
Chayote, raw	5	102
Cheese, natural & processed, cheese foods, cheese spreads:		
Natural cheeses:		
Blue or Roquefort type	NA	NA
Brick	NA	NA
Camembert (domestic)	NA	111
Cheddar (domestic type, commonly called American)	700	82
Cottage (large or small curd):		
Creamed	229	85
Uncreamed	290	72
Cream	250	74
Limburger	NA	NA
Parmesan	734	149

*Estimated average based on the addition of salt in the amount of 0.6 percent of the finished product.

	SODIUM (MG PER 3.5 OZ OR 100 G)	POTASSIUM (MG PER 3.5 OZ OR 100 G)
Cheese continued		
Swiss (domestic)	710	104
Pasteurized process cheese:		
American	1,136*	80
Pimiento (American)	NA	NA
Swiss	1,167*	100
Pasteurized process cheese food, American	NA	NA
Pasteurized process cheese spread, American	1,625*	240
Cheese fondue, from home recipe	542	165
Cheese soufflé, from home recipe	364	121
Cheese straws	721	65
Cherries:		
Raw:		
Sour, red	2	191
Sweet	2	191
Candied	NA	NA
Canned:		
Sour, red, solids & liquid:		
Water pack	2	130
Syrup pack:		
Light	1	126
Sweet, solids & liquid:		
Water pack	1	130
Syrup pack:		
Light	1	128
Frozen, not thawed:		
Sour, red:		
Unsweetened	2	188
Sweetened	2	130
Cherries, maraschino, bottled, solids & liquid	NA	NA
Chestnuts:		
Fresh	6	454
Dried	12	875
Chewing gum	NA	NA
Chicken:		
All classes:		
Light meat without skin:		
Cooked, roasted	64	151
Dark meat without skin:		
Cooked, roasted	86	321

*Estimated average based on the addition of salt in the amount of 0.6 percent of the finished product.

	SODIUM (MG PER 3.5 OZ OR 100 G)	POTASSIUM (MG PER 3.5 OZ OR 100 G)
Chicken continued		
Broilers, flesh only, cooked, broiled	66	274
Fryers:		
Flesh & skin:		
Cooked, fried	NA	NA
Flesh only:		
Cooked, fried	78	38
Light meat with skin:		
Cooked, fried	NA	NA
Dark meat with skin:		
Cooked, fried	NA	NA
Light meat without skin:		
Cooked, fried	68	434
Dark meat without skin:		
Cooked, fried	88	330
Roasters:		
Flesh only:		
Cooked, roasted	77	376
Light meat without skin:		
Cooked, roasted	66	422
Dark meat without skin:		
Cooked, roasted	88	330
Hens & cocks:		
Flesh only:		
Cooked, stewed	55	272
Light meat without skin:		
Cobked, stewed	48	306
Dark meat without skin:		
Cooked, stewed	64	239
Chicken, canned, meat only, boned	NA	138
Chicken à la king, cooked from home recipe	310	165
Chicken fricassee, cooked from home recipe	154	140
Chicken pot pie:		
Home-prepared, baked	256	148
Commercial, frozen, unheated	411	153
Chicken & noodles, cooked, from home recipe	250	62
Chick-peas or garbanzos, mature seeds, dry, raw	26	797

46

	SODIUM (MG PER 3.5 OZ OR 100 G)	POTASSIUM (MG PER 3.5 OZ OR 100 G)
Chicory, witloof (also called French or Belgian endive), bleached head (forced), raw	7	182
Chicory greens, raw	NA	420
Chili con carne, canned:		
With beans	531	233
Without beans	NA	NA
Chives, raw	NA	250
Chocolate:		
Bitter or baking	4	830
Bittersweet. See candy.		
Chocolate syrup:		
Thin type	52	282
Fudge type	89	284
Chop suey, with meat:		
Cooked, from home recipe	421	170
Canned	551	138
Chow mein, chicken (without noodles):		
Cooked, from home recipe	287	189
Canned	290	167
Clams, raw:		
Soft:		
Meat & liquid	NA	NA
Meat only	36	235
Hard or round:		
Meat & liquid	NA	NA
Meat only	205	311
Hard, soft & unspecified:		
Meat & liquid	NA	NA
Meat only	120	181
Clams, canned, including hard, soft, razor & unspecified:		
Solids & liquid	NA	140
Clam fritters (prepared with flour, baking powder, butter, eggs)	NA	147
Cocoa & chocolate-flavored beverage powders:		
Cocoa powder with nonfat dry milk	525	800
Cocoa powder without milk	268	500
Milk for hot chocolate (values apply to products w/o added vitamins & minerals)	382	605

47

	SODIUM (MG PER 3.5 OZ OR 100 G)	POTASSIUM (MG PER 3.5 OZ OR 100 G)
Cocoa, dry powder:		
High-fat or breakfast:		
Plain	6	1,522
Medium-fat:		
High-medium fat:		
Plain	6	1,522
Low-medium fat:		
Plain	6	1,522
Low fat:	6	1,522
Coconut meat:		
Fresh	23	256
Dried:		
Unsweetened	NA	588
Sweetened, shredded	NA	353
Cod:		
Cooked, broiled	110	407
Canned	NA	NA
Dehydrated, lightly salted	8,100	160
Dried, salted	NA	NA
Codfish cakes. See Fishcakes.		
Coffee, instant, water-soluble solids:		
Dry powder	72	3,250
Beverage	1	36
Coleslaw, made with:		
French dressing (homemade)	131	197
French dressing (commercial)	268	205
Mayonnaise	120	199
Salad dressing (mayonnaise type)	124	192
Collards:		
Cooked, boiled, drained:		
Leaves without stems, cooked in:		
Small amount of water	NA	262
Large amount of water	NA	243
Leaves, including stems, cooked in:		
Small amount of water	25	234
Frozen:		
Cooked, boiled, drained	16	236

48

	SODIUM (MG PER 3.5 OZ OR 100 G)	POTASSIUM (MG PER 3.5 OZ OR 100 G)
Cookies:		
Assorted, packaged, commercial	365	67
Brownies with nuts:		
Baked from home recipe, enriched flour	251	190
Frozen, with chocolate icing, commercial	200	179
Butter, thin, rich	418	60
Chocplate	137	128
Chocolate chip:		
Baked from home recipe, enriched flour	348	117
Commercial type	401	134
Coconut bars	148	228
Fig bars	252	198
Gingersnaps	571	462
Ladyfingers	71	71
Macaroons	34	463
Marshmallow	209	91
Molasses	386	138
Oatmeal with raisins	162	370
Peanut	173	175
Raisin	52	272
Sandwich type	483	38
Shortbread	60	66
Sugar, soft thick, with enriched flour, home recipe	318	76
Sugar wafers	189	60
Vanilla wafers	252	72
Cookie mixes & cookies baked from mixes:		
Brownie, with enriched flour:		
Complete mix:		
Brownies made with water, nuts	218	180
Incomplete mix:		
Brownies, made with egg, water, nuts	166	168
Plain, with unenriched flour:		
Cookies, made with egg, water	347	42
Cookies, made with milk	345	42

	SODIUM (MG PER 3.5 OZ OR 100 G)	POTASSIUM (MG PER 3.5 OZ OR 100 G)
Cookies continued		
Cookie dough, plain, chilled in roll:		
Baked	548	48
Corn, sweet:		
Cooked, boiled, drained, white & yellow:		
Kernels, cut off cob before cooking	Trace	165
Kernels, cooked on cob	Trace	196
Canned:		
Regular pack:		
Cream style, white & yellow:		
Solids & liquid	236*	(97)
Whole kernel:		
Vacuum pack, yellow:		
Solids & liquid	236*	(97)
Wet pack, white & yellow:		
Solids & liquid	236	97
Drained solids	236	97
Special dietary pack (low-sodium):		
Cream style, white & yellow:		
Solids & liquid	2	(97)
Whole kernel, wet pack, white & yellow:		
Solids & liquid	2	97
Drained solids	2	97
Frozen:		
Kernels, cut off cob		
Cooked, boiled, drained	1	184
Kernels, on cob		
Cooked, boiled, drained	1	231
Corn flour	(1)	NA
Corn fritters	477	133
Corn grits, degermed:		
Enriched:		
Cooked	205	11
Unenriched:		
Cooked	205	11
Corn products used mainly as ready-to-eat breakfast cereals:		

*Estimated average based on the addition of salt in the amount of 0.6 percent of the finished product.

	SODIUM (MG PER 3.5 OZ OR 100 G)	POTASSIUM (MG PER 3.5 OZ OR 100 G)
Corn products continued		
Corn flakes:		
Added nutrients	1,005	120
Added nutrients, sugar-covered	775	NA
Corn, puffed:		
Added nutrients	1,060	NA
Presweetened:		
Added nutrients	300	NA
Cocoa-flavored, added nutrients	850	NA
Fruit-flavored, added nutrients	600	NA
Corn, shredded, added nutrients	988	NA
Corn, rice, & wheat flakes, mixed, added nutrients	950	NA
Corn, flaked, with protein concentrate (casein) & other added nutrients	1,100	NA
Corn pudding	436	169
Cornbread, baked from home recipes:		
Cornbread, southern style, made with:		
Whole-ground cornmeal	628	157
Degermed cornmeal, enriched	591	157
Johnnycake (northern style cornbread), made with enriched, yellow degermed cornmeal	690	188
Corn pone, made with white, whole-ground cornmeal	396	61
Spoonbread, made with white whole-ground cornmeal	482	152
Cornbread baked from mix:		
Cornbread, made with egg, milk	744	127
Cornmeal, white or yellow:		
Degermed, enriched:		
Cooked	110	16
Degermed, unenriched:		
Cooked	110	16

	SODIUM (MG PER 3.5 OZ OR 100 G)	POTASSIUM (MG PER 3.5 OZ OR 100 G)
Cornmeal continued		
Self-rising:		
Whole-ground:		
With soft wheat flour added	1,380	212*
Without wheat flour added	1,380	234*
Degermed:		
With soft wheat flour added	1,380	109
Without wheat flour added	1,380	113
Corn salad, raw	NA	NA
Cornstarch	Trace	Trace
Cottonseed flour	NA	NA
Cowpeas, including blackeye peas:		
Immature seeds:		
Cooked, boiled, drained	1	379
Canned, solids & liquid	236†	352†
Frozen (blackeye peas only):		
Cooked, boiled, drained	39	337
Young pods, with seeds:		
Cooked, boiled, drained	3	196
Mature seeds, dry:		
Cooked	8	229
Crab, including blue, Dungeness, rock & king cooked, steamed	NA	NA
Crab, canned	1,000	110
Crab, deviled (prepared with bread cubes, butter, parsley, eggs, lemon juice & catsup)	867	166
Crab imperial (prepared with butter, flour, milk, onion, green pepper, eggs & lemon juice)	728	131
Crackers:		
Animal	303	95
Butter	1,092	113
Cheese	1,039	100
Graham:		
Chocolate-coated	407	320
Plain	670	384
Sugar-honey coated	504	270
Saltines	(1,100)	(120)

*Amount of potassium contributed by cornmeal and flour. Small quantities of additional potassium may be provided by other ingredients.
†Estimated average based on the addition of salt in the amount of 0.6 percent of the finished product.

	SODIUM (MG PER 3.5 OZ OR 100 G)	POTASSIUM (MG PER 3.5 OZ OR 100 G)
Crackers continued		
Sandwich type, peanut-cheese	992	226
Soda	1,100	120
Whole-wheat	547	NA
Cracker meal. See Crackers, soda.		
Cranberries:		
Raw	2	82
Dehydrated, uncooked	16	644
Cranberry juice cocktail, bottled	1	10
Cranberry sauce, sweetened:		
Canned, strained	1	30
Home-prepared, unstrained	1	38
Cranberry-orange relish, uncooked	1	72
Crayfish, freshwater, & spiny lobster; raw	NA	NA
Cream, fluid:		
Half-and-half (cream & milk)	46	129
Light, coffee or table	43	122
Light whipping	36	102
Heavy whipping	32	89
Cream substitutes, dried, containing:		
Cream, skim milk (calcium reduced) lactose	575	NA
Cream, skim milk lactose & sodium hexametaphosphate	NA	NA
Cream puffs with custard filling	83	121
Croaker, Atlantic:		
Cooked, baked	120	323
Cucumbers, raw:		
Not pared	6	160
Pared	6	160
Custard, baked	79	146
Dandelion greens:		
Cooked, boiled, drained	44	236
Dates, domestic, natural & dry	1	648
Doughnuts:		
Cake type	501	90
Yeast-leavened	234	80
Duck, domesticated, raw:		
Total edible	NA	NA
Duck, wild, raw:		
Total edible	NA	NA

	SODIUM (MG PER 3.5 OZ OR 100 G)	POTASSIUM (MG PER 3.5 OZ OR 100 G)
Eclairs with custard filling & chocolate icing	82	122
Eel, American, raw	NA	NA
Eel, smoked	NA	NA
Eggs:		
Chicken:		
Raw:		
Whole, fresh & frozen	122	129
Whites, fresh & frozen	146	139
Yolks, fresh	52	98
Yolks, frozen	63	100
Yolks, frozen, sugared	57	91
Cooked:		
Fried	338	140
Hard-boiled	122	129
Omelet	257	146
Poached	271	128
Scrambled	257	146
Dried:		
Whole	427	463
Whole, stabilized (glucose reduced)	444	482
White, flakes	1,033	937
White, powder	1,103	1,000
Yolk	100	186
Duck, whole, fresh, raw	(122)	(129)
Goose, whole, fresh, raw	NA	NA
Turkey, whole, fresh, raw	NA	NA
Eggplant:		
Cooked, boiled, drained	1	150
Endive (curly endive & escarole), raw	14	294
Escarole, raw. See endive.		
Farina:		
Enriched:		
Regular:		
Cooked	144	9
Quick-cooking:		
Cooked	190	10
Instant cooking:		
Cooked	188	13
Unenriched, regular:		
Cooked	144	9

	SODIUM (MG PER 3.5 OZ OR 100 G)	POTASSIUM (MG PER 3.5 OZ OR 100 G)
Fats, cooking (vegetable fat)	0	0
Fennel, common, leaves, raw	NA	397
Figs:		
Raw	2	194
Candied	NA	NA
Canned, solids & liquid:		
Syrup pack:		
Light	2	152
Dried, uncooked	34	640
Filberts (hazelnuts)	2	704
Finnan haddie (smoked haddock)	NA	NA
Fish cakes, cooked:		
Fried (prepared with canned flaked fish, potato & egg)	NA	NA
Frozen, fried, reheated	NA	NA
Fish flakes, canned	NA	NA
Fish loaf, cooked (prepared with canned flaked fish, bread cubes, eggs, tomatoes, onion & fat)	NA	NA
Fish sticks, frozen, cooked	NA	NA
Flatfishes (flounders, soles & sanddabs), raw	78	342
Flounder, cooked, baked	237	587
Flour. See Corn, Rice, Rye, Soya, Wheat.		
Frog legs, raw	NA	NA
Fruit cocktail, canned, solids & liquid:		
Water pack, with or without artificial sweetener	5	168
Syrup pack:		
Light	5	164
Fruit salad, canned solids & liquid:		
Water pack, with or without artificial sweetener	1	139
Syrup pack:		
Light	1	136
Garbanzos. See Chickpeas.		
Garlic, cloves, raw	19	529
Gelatin, dry	NA	NA
Gelatin dessert powder & desserts made from dessert powder:		
Dessert powder	318	NA

	SODIUM (MG PER 3.5 OZ OR 100 G)	POTASSIUM (MG PER 3.5 OZ OR 100 G)
Gelatin continued		
Desserts, made with water:		
Plain	51	NA
With fruit added	34	NA
Gingerroot, crystallized (candied)	NA	NA
Gingerroot, fresh	6	26
Gizzard:		
Chicken, all classes:		
Cooked, simmered	57	21
Turkey, all classes:		
Cooked, simmered	51	14
Goose, domesticated:		
Total edible:		
Cooked, roasted	NA	NA
Flesh & skin:		
Cooked, roasted	NA	NA
Flesh only:		
Cooked, roasted	124	605
Gooseberries:		
Canned, solids & liquids:		
Water pack, with or without artificial sweetener	1	105
Syrup pack:		
Heavy	1	98
Grapefruit (all varieties):		
Raw:		
Pulp:		
Pink, red, white	1	135
Juice:		
Pink, red, white	1	162
Canned:		
Segments, solids & liquids:		
Water pack, with or without artificial sweetener	4	144
Syrup pack	1	135
Juice:		
Unsweetened	1	162
Sweetened	1	162
Frozen concentrated juice:		
Unsweetened:		
Diluted with 3 parts water, by volume	1	170
Sweetened:		
Diluted with 3 parts water, by volume	1	144

	SODIUM (MG PER 3.5 OZ OR 100 G)	POTASSIUM (MG PER 3.5 OZ OR 100 G)
Grapefruit juice & orange juice blended:		
Canned:		
Unsweetened	1	184
Sweetened	1	184
Frozen concentrate, unsweetened:		
Diluted with 3 parts water, by volume	Trace	177
Grapefruit peel, candied	NA	NA
Grapes:		
Raw:		
American type (slip skin) as Concord, Delaware, Niagara, Catawba & Scuppernong	3	158
European type (adherent skin) as Malaga, Muscat, Thompson Seedless, Emperor & Flame Tokay	3	173
Canned:		
Thompson Seedless, solids & liquid:		
Water pack, with or without artificial sweetener	4	110
Syrup pack, heavy	4	105
Grape juice:		
Canned or bottled	2	116
Frozen concentrate, sweetened:		
Diluted with 3 parts water, by volume	1	34
Grouper, including red, black, & speckled hind; raw	NA	NA
Haddock:		
Cooked, fried (dipped in egg, milk & breadcrumbs)	177	348
Smoked, canned or not canned	NA	NA
Hake, including Pacific hake, squirrel hake, and silver hake or whiting; raw.	74	363
Halibut, Atlantic & Pacific:		
Cooked, broiled	134	525
Smoked	NA	NA
Ham croquette	342	83

	SODIUM (MG PER 3.5 OZ OR 100 G)	POTASSIUM (MG PER 3.5 OZ OR 100 G)
Herring (Lake herring):		
Raw:		
Atlantic	NA	NA
Pacific	74	420
Canned, solids & liquid:		
Plain	NA	NA
In tomato sauce	NA	NA
Pickled, Bismarck type	NA	NA
Salted or brined	NA	NA
Smoked:		
Bloaters	NA	NA
Hard	6,231	157
Kippered	NA	NA
Honey, strained or extracted	5	51
Honeydew melon. See Muskmelons.		
Horseradish, prepared	96	290
Ice cream & frozen custard (commercial products, without added salt):		
Regular:		
Approximately 10% fat	63	181
Approximately 12% fat	40	112
Rich, approximately 16% fat	33	95
Ice cream cones	232	244
Ice milk	68	195
Ices, water, lime	Traces	3
Jack, mackerel, raw	NA	NA
Jams & preserves	12	88
Kale:		
Cooked, boiled, drained:		
Leaves, without stems, midribs	(43)	(221)
Leaves, including stems	43	221
Frozen:		
Cooked, boiled, drained	21	193
Kidneys:		
Beef:		
Cooked, braised	253	324
Kingfish; southern, gulf, & northern (whiting); raw	83	250
Kohlrabi, thickened bulb-like stems:		
Cooked, boiled, drained	6	260

	SODIUM (MG PER 3.5 OZ OR 100 G)	POTASSIUM (MG PER 3.5 OZ OR 100 G)
Kumquats, raw	7	236
Lake herring (cisco), raw	47	319
Lake trout, raw	NA	NA
Lake trout (siscowet), raw	NA	NA
Lamb:		
Retail cuts, trimmed to retail level:		
Leg:		
Prime grade:		
Total edible:		
Cooked, roasted	70	290
Choice, grade:		
Total edible:		
Cooked, roasted	70	290
Good grade:		
Total edible:		
Cooked, roasted	70	290
Loin:		
Prime grade:		
Total edible:		
Cooked, broiled chops	70	290
Choice grade:		
Total edible:		
Cooked, broiled chops	70	290
Good grade:		
Total edible:		
Cooked, broiled chops	70	290
Rib:		
Prime grade:		
Total edible:		
Cooked, broiled chops	70	290
Choice grade:		
Total edible:		
Cooked, broiled chops	70	290
Good grade:		
Total edible:		
Cooked, broiled chops	70	290
Shoulder:		
Prime grade:		
Total edible:		
Cooked, roasted	70	290
Choice grade:		
Total edible:		
Cooked, roasted	70	290

	SODIUM (MG PER 3.5 OZ OR 100 G)	POTASSIUM (MG PER 3.5 OZ OR 100 G)
Lamb continued		
Good grade:		
Total edible:		
Cooked, roasted	70	290
Lambsquarters:		
Cooked, boiled, drained	NA	NA
Lard	0	0
Lemons, raw:		
Peeled fruit	2	138
Fruit, including peel	3	145
Lemon juice:		
Raw	1	141
Canned or bottled, unsweetened	1	141
Frozen, unsweetened:		
Single-strength juice	1	141
Concentrate	5	658
Lemon peel:		
Raw	6	160
Candied	NA	NA
Lemonade concentrate, frozen:		
Diluted with 4⅓ parts water, by volume	Trace	6
Lentils, mature seeds, dry:		
Whole:		
Cooked	NA	249
Split, without seed coat, raw	NA	NA
Lettuce, raw:		
Butterhead varieties, such as Boston types & Bibb	9	264
Cos, or romaine, such as Dark Green & White Paris	9	264
Crisphead varieties, such as Iceberg, New York, & Great Lake strains	9	175
Looseleaf or bunching varieties, such as Grand Rapids, Salad Bowl, & Simpson	9	264
Lime juice:		
Raw	1	104
Canned or bottled, unsweetened	1	104
Limeade concentrate, frozen:		
Diluted with 4⅓ parts water, by volume	Trace	13

	SODIUM (MG PER 3.5 OZ OR 100 G)	POTASSIUM (MG PER 3.5 OZ OR 100 G)
Liver:		
Beef:		
Cooked, fried	184	380
Calf:		
Cooked, fried	118	453
Chicken, all classes:		
Cooked, simmered	61	151
Hog:		
Cooked, fried	111	395
Lamb:		
Cooked, broiled	85	331
Turkey, all classes:		
Cooked, simmered	55	141
Lobster, northern:		
Canned or cooked	210	180
Lobster Newburg (prepared with butter, egg yolks, sherry & cream)	229	171
Lobster Salad (prepared with onion, sweet pickle, celery, eggs, mayonnaise & tomatoes)	124	264
Loganberries:		
Raw	(1)	170
Canned, solids & liquid:		
Water pack, with or without artificial sweetener	1	115
Juice pack	1	170
Syrup pack:		
Light	1	111
Macadamia nuts	NA	264
Macaroni:		
Enriched:		
Cooked, firm stage (8–10 min.)	1	79
Cooked, tender stage (14–20 min.)	1	61
Unenriched:		
Cooked, firm stage (8–10 min.)	1	79
Cooked, tender stage (14–20 min.)	1	61
Macaroni & cheese:		
Baked; made from home recipe (enriched macaroni)	543	120

	SODIUM (MG PER 3.5 OZ OR 100 G)	POTASSIUM (MG PER 3.5 OZ OR 100 G)
Macaroni continued		
Canned	304	58
Mackerel:		
Salted	NA	NA
Smoked	NA	NA
Mackerel, Atlantic:		
Canned, solids & liquid	NA	NA
Cooked, broiled with butter or margarine	NA	NA
Mackerel, Pacific:		
Canned, solids & liquid	NA	NA
Mangos, raw	7	189
Marmalade, citrus	987	23
Marmalade plums. See Sapotes.	14	33
Milk, cow:		
Fluid (pasteurized & raw):		
Whole:		
3.5% fat	50	144
3.7% fat (national average for milk on the farm production basis)	50	140
Skim	52	145
Partially skimmed with 2% nonfat milk solids added	61	175
Half-and-half (cream & milk). See cream		
Canned:		
Evaporated (unsweetened)	118	303
Condensed (sweetened)	112	314
Dry:		
Whole	405	1,330
Skim (nonfat solids), regular	532	1,795
Skim (nonfat solids), instant	526	1,725
Malted:		
Dry powder (unfortified)	440	720
Beverage (prepared with malted milk powder & whole milk)	91	200
Chocolate drink, fluid, commercial:		
Made with skim milk	46	142
Made with whole (3.5% fat) milk	47	146
Chocolate beverages, homemade:		
Hot chocolate	48	148

	SODIUM (MG PER 3.5 OZ OR 100 G)	POTASSIUM (MG PER 3.5 OZ OR 100 G)
Milk continued		
Hot cocoa	51	145
Buttermilk. See Buttermilk.		
Milk, goat, fluid	34	180
Milk, human, U.S. samples	16	51
Molasses, cane:		
Light	15	917
Medium	37	1,063
Blackstrap	96	2,927
Barbados	NA	NA
Muffins, baked from home recipes:		
Plain, made with:		
Enriched flour	441	125
Unenriched flour	441	125
Other, made with enriched flour:		
Blueberry	632	115
Bran	448	431
Corn, made with:		
Enriched degermed cornmeal	481	135
Whole-ground cornmeal	495	132
Muffins baked from mixes (contain yellow degermed cornmeal):		
Muffins, made with egg, milk	479	110
Muffins, made with egg, water	346	104
Mushrooms:		
Raw	15	414
Canned, solids & liquid	400	197
Muskmelons:		
Raw:		
Cantaloups, other netted varieties	12	251
Casaba (Golden Beauty)	(12)	(251)
Honeydew	12	251
Frozen:		
Melon balls (cantaloupe & honeydew) in syrup, not thawed	9	188
Mussels, Atlantic & Pacific, raw:		
Meat & liquid	NA	NA
Meat only	289	315
Mussels, Pacific, canned, drained solids	NA	NA
Mustard greens:		
Cooked, boiled, drained	18	220

	SODIUM (MG PER 3.5 OZ OR 100 G)	POTASSIUM (MG PER 3.5 OZ OR 100 G)
Mustard greens continued		
Frozen:		
Cooked, boiled, drained	10	157
Mustard spinach (tendergreen):		
Cooked, boiled, drained	NA	NA
Mustard, prepared:		
Brown	1,307	130
Yellow	1,252	130
Noodles, egg noodles:		
Enriched:		
Cooked	2	44
Unenriched:		
Cooked	2	44
Noodles, chow mein, canned	NA	NA
Oat products used mainly as hot breakfast cereals:		
Oat cereal with toasted wheat germ & soy grits:		
Cooked	292	Trace
Oat flakes, maple-flavored, instant-cooking:		
Cooked	107	NA
Oat granules, maple-flavored, quick-cooking:		
Cooked	72	NA
Oat & wheat cereal:		
Cooked	168	NA
Oatmeal or rolled oats:		
Cooked	218	61
Oat products used mainly as ready-to-eat breakfast cereals:		
Oats, shredded, with protein & other added nutrients	610	NA
Oats (with or without corn), puffed, added nutrients	1,267	NA
Oats (with or without corn, wheat), puffed, added nutrients, sugar-covered	588	NA
Oats (with soy flour & rice), flaked, added nutrients	1,200	NA
Ocean perch, Atlantic (redfish):		
Cooked, fried (dipped in egg, milk & bread crumbs)	153	284
Frozen, breaded, fried, reheated	NA	NA
Oils, salad or cooking	0	0

	SODIUM (MG PER 3.5 OZ OR 100 G)	POTASSIUM (MG PER 3.5 OZ OR 100 G)
Okra:		
Cooked, boiled, drained	2	174
Frozen, cuts & pods:		
Cooked, boiled, drained	2	164
Olives, pickled; canned or bottled:		
Green	2,400	55
Ripe:		
Ascolano (extra large, mammoth, giant, jumbo)	813	34
Manzanilla (small, medium, large, extra large)	813	34
Mission (small, medium, large, extra large)	750	27
Sevillano (giant, jumbo, colossal, super colossal)	828	44
Ripe, salt-cured, oil-coated, Greek style	3,288	NA
Onions, mature (dry):		
Raw	10	157
Cooked, boiled, drained	7	110
Dehydrated, flaked	88	138
Onions, young green (bunching varieties), raw:		
Bulb & entire top	5	23
Oranges, raw:		
Peeled fruit:		
All commercial varieties	1	200
Orange juice:		
Raw:		
All commercial varieties	1	200
Canned:		
Unsweetened	1	199
Sweetened	1	(199)
Canned concentrate, unsweetened:		
Diluted with 5 parts water, by volume	1	192
Frozen concentrate, unsweetened:		
Diluted with 3 parts water, by volume	1	186
Orange juice & apricot juice drink, canned	Trace	94
Orange peel:		
Raw	3	212

	SODIUM (MG PER 3.5 OZ OR 100 G)	POTASSIUM (MG PER 3.5 OZ OR 100 G)
Orange peel continued		
Candied	NA	NA
Oysters:		
Raw, meat only:		
Eastern	73	121
Pacific & western (Olympia)	NA	NA
Cooked, fried (dipped in egg, milk & bread crumbs)	206	203
Canned, solids & liquid	NA	70
Frozen, solids & liquid	380	210
Oyster stew:		
Commercial, frozen:		
Condensed	680	205
Prepared with equal volume of water	340	102
Prepared with equal volume of milk	366	176
Home-prepared (contains added salt & butter):		
1 part oysters to 2 parts milk by volume	339	133
1 part oysters to 3 parts milk by volume	203	138
Pancakes, baked from home recipe, made with:		
Enriched flour	425	123
Unenriched flour	425	123
Pancake & waffle baked from mixes:		
Plain & buttermilk:		
Mix (pancake & waffle), with enriched flour, dry form	1,433	162
Pancakes:		
Made with milk	451	156
Made with egg, milk	564	154
Mix (pancake & waffle) with unenriched flour, dry form		
Pancakes:		
Made with milk	451	156
Made with egg, milk	564	154
Buckwheat & other cereal flours:		
Mix, dry form	1,334	476

	SODIUM (MG PER 3.5 OZ OR 100 G)	POTASSIUM (MG PER 3.5 OZ OR 100 G)
Pancakes continued		
Pancakes, made with egg, milk	464	245
Papayas, raw	3	234
Parsley, common garden (plain) & curled-leaf varieties, raw	45	727
Parsnips:		
Cooked, boiled, drained	8	379
Pastinas, enriched, dry form:		
Egg	5	NA
Vegetable	NA	NA
Spinach	NA	NA
Pâté de foi gras, canned	NA	NA
Peaches:		
Raw	1	202
Canned, solids & liquid:		
Water pack, with or without artificial sweetener	2	137
Juice pack	2	205
Syrup:		
Light	2	133
Dehydrated, sulfured, nugget-type & pieces:		
Uncooked	(21)	(1,229)
Cooked, fruit & liquid, with added sugar	(5)	(292)
Dried, sulfured:		
Uncooked	16	950
Cooked, fruit & liquid:		
Without added sugar	5	297
With added sugar	4	261
Frozen, sliced, sweetened, not thawed	2	124
Peach nectar, canned	1	78
Peanuts:		
Raw, without skins	5	674
Boiled	4	462
Roasted, with skins	5	701
Roasted & salted	418	674
Peanut butters made with:		
Small amounts of added fat, salt	607	670
Small amounts of added fat, sweetener, salt	606	652

	SODIUM (MG PER 3.5 OZ OR 100 G)	POTASSIUM (MG PER 3.5 OZ OR 100 G)
Peanut Butters continued		
Moderate amounts of added fat, sweetener, salt	605	627
Peanut spread	597	530
Peanut flour, defatted	9	1,186
Pears:		
Raw, including skin	2	130
Candied	NA	NA
Canned, solids & liquid:		
Water pack, with or without artificial sweetener	1	88
Juice pack	1	130
Syrup pack:		
Light	1	85
Dried, sulfured:		
Uncooked	7	573
Cooked, fruit & liquid:		
Without added sugar	3	269
With added sugar	3	244
Pear nectar, canned	1	39
Peas, green, immature:		
Raw	2	316
Cooked, boiled, drained	1	196
Canned:		
Regular pack:		
Solids & liquid	236*	96
Drained solids	236*	96
Special dietary pack (low-sodium):		
Solids & liquid	3	96
Drained solids	3	96
Sweet (sweet wrinkled peas, sugar peas):		
Regular pack:		
Solids & liquid	236*	96
Drained solids	236*	96
Special dietary pack (low-sodium):		
Solids & liquid	3	96
Drained solids	3	96
Frozen:		
Cooked, boiled, drained	115	135

*Estimated average based on the addition of salt in the amount of 0.6 percent of the finished product.

	SODIUM (MG PER 3.5 OZ OR 100 G)	POTASSIUM (MG PER 3.5 OZ OR 100 G)
Peas, mature seeds, dry:		
Whole:		
Raw	35	1,005
Split, without seed coat:		
Cooked (unsalted)	13	296
Peas & carrots, frozen:		
Cooked, boiled, drained	84	157
Pecans	Trace	603
Peppers, hot, chili:		
Immature, green:		
Canned:		
Pods, excluding seeds; solids & liquid	NA	NA
Chili sauce	NA	NA
Mature, red:		
Raw:		
Pods, excluding seeds	25	564
Canned, chili sauce	NA	NA
Dried:		
Pods	373	120
Chili powder with added seasoning	1,574	102
Peppers, sweet, garden varieties:		
Immature, green:		
Raw	13	213
Cooked:		
Boiled, drained	9	149
Stuffed with beef & crumbs	314	258
Mature, red, raw	NA	NA
Perch, white, raw	NA	NA
Perch, yellow, raw	68	230
Persimmons, raw (Native)	1	310
Pheasant, raw:		
Total edible	NA	NA
Flesh & skin	NA	NA
Pickles:		
Cucumber:		
Dill	1,428	200
Fresh (as bread-and-butter pickles)	673	NA
Sour	1,353	NA
Sweet	NA	NA

	SODIUM (MG PER 3.5 OZ OR 100 G)	POTASSIUM (MG PER 3.5 OZ OR 100 G)
Pickles continued		
Chowchow (cucumber with added cauliflower, onion, mustard):		
Sour	1,338	NA
Sweet	527	NA
Relish, finely cut or chopped:		
Sour	NA	NA
Sweet	712	NA
Pies:		
Baked, pie crust made with unenriched flour:		
Apple	301	80
Banana custard	194	203
Blackberry	268	100
Blueberry	268	65
Boston Cream. See Cakes.		
Butterscotch	214	95
Cherry	304	105
Chocolate chiffon	252	110
Chocolate meringue	256	139
Coconut custard	247	163
Custard	287	137
Lemon chiffon	261	81
Lemon meringue	282	50
Mince	448	178
Peach	268	149
Pecan	221	123
Pineapple	271	72
Pineapple chiffon	256	98
Pineapple custard	186	97
Pumpkin	214	160
Raisin	285	192
Rhubarb	270	159
Strawberry	194	120
Sweet potato	218	163
Frozen in baked form:		
Apple	213	72
Cherry	229	82
Coconut custard	252	172
Pie baked from mix, coconut custard:		
Pie prepared with egg yolk & milk	235	154

	SODIUM (MG PER 3.5 OZ OR 100 G)	POTASSIUM (MG PER 3.5 OZ OR 100 G)
Pie crust or plain pastry baked with:		
Enriched flour	611	50
Unenriched flour	611	50
Pie crust baked from mix (including stick form):		
Pie crust, prepared with water	813	50
Pimientos, canned, solids & liquid	NA	NA
Pineapple:		
Raw	1	146
Candied	NA	NA
Canned, solids & liquid:		
Water pack, all styles, except crushed, with or without artificial sweetener	1	99
Juice pack, all styles	1	147
Syrup pack, all styles:		
Light	1	97
Frozen chunks, sweetened, not thawed	2	100
Pineapple juice:		
Canned, unsweetened	1	149
Frozen concentrate, unsweetened:		
Diluted with 3 parts water, by volume	1	136
Pineapple juice & grapefruit juice drink, canned	Trace	62
Pineapple juice & orange juice drink, canned	Trace	70
Pinenuts:		
Pignolias (Piñon)	NA	NA
Pistachio nuts	NA	972
Pizza, with cheese:		
From home recipe (unenriched flour), baked:		
With cheese topping	702	130
With sausage topping	729	168
Frozen:		
Baked	647	114
Plantain (baking banana), raw	5	385
Plate dinners, frozen, commercial, unheated:		

	SODIUM (MG PER 3.5 OZ OR 100 G)	POTASSIUM (MG PER 3.5 OZ OR 100 G)
Plate dinners continued		
Beef pot roast; whole oven-browned potatoes; peas & corn	259	244
Chicken, fried; mashed potatoes; mixed vegetables (carrots, peas, corn, beans)	344	112
Meatloaf with tomato sauce, mashed potatoes & peas	393	115
Turkey, sliced; mashed potatoes; peas	400	176
Plums:		
Raw:		
Damson	2	299
Prune-type	1	170
Canned, solids & liquid:		
Purple (Italian prunes):		
Water pack, with or without artificial sweetener	2	148
Syrup pack:		
Light	1	145
Pollock, cooked, creamed (prepared with flour, butter, milk)	111	238
Popcorn:		
Popped:		
Plain	(3)	NA
Oil & salt added	1,940	NA
Sugar-coated (without added salt)	1	NA
Popovers, baked (from home recipe with enriched flour)	220	150
Pork, fresh:		
Composite of trimmed lean cuts, ham, loin, shoulder & spare ribs:		
Fat class:		
Total edible:		
Cooked, roasted	65	390
Separable lean:		
Cooked, roasted	65	390
Medium-fat class:		
Total edible:		
Cooked, roasted	65	390

	SODIUM (MG PER 3.5 OZ OR 100 G)	POTASSIUM (MG PER 3.5 OZ OR 100 G)
Pork continued		
Separable lean:		
Cooked, roasted	65	390
Thin class:		
Total edible:		
Cooked, roasted	65	390
Separable lean:		
Cooked, roasted	65	390
Retail cuts, trimmed to retail level:		
Ham:		
Fat class:		
Total edible:		
Cooked, roasted	65	390
Medium-fat class:		
Total edible:		
Cooked, roasted	65	390
Thin class:		
Total edible:		
Cooked, roasted	65	390
Loin:		
Fat class:		
Total edible:		
Cooked, roasted	65	390
Cooked, broiled	65	390
Medium-fat class:		
Total edible:		
Cooked, roasted	65	390
Cooked, broiled	65	390
Thin class:		
Total edible:		
Cooked, roasted	65	390
Cooked, broiled	65	390
Boston butt:		
Fat class:		
Total edible:		
Cooked, roasted	65	390
Medium-fat class:		
Total edible:		
Cooked, roasted	65	390
Thin class:		
Total edible:		
Cooked, roasted	65	390

	SODIUM (MG PER 3.5 OZ OR 100 G)	POTASSIUM (MG PER 3.5 OZ OR 100 G)
Pork continued		
Picnic:		
Fat class:		
Total edible:		
Cooked, simmered	65	390
Medium-fat class:		
Total edible:		
Cooked, simmered	65	390
Thin class:		
Total edible:		
Cooked, simmered	65	390
Spareribs:		
Fat class:		
Total edible		
Cooked, braised	65	390
Medium-fat class:		
Total edible:		
Cooked, braised	65	390
Thin class:		
Total edible:		
Cooked, braised	65	390
Pork, cured:		
Dry, long-cure, country-style ham	65	390
Light-cure, commercial:		
Ham, medium-fat class:		
Cooked, roasted	65	390
Boston butt, medium-fat class:		
Cooked, roasted	65	390
Picnic, medium-fat class		
Cooked, roasted	65	390
Pork, cured, canned:		
Ham, contents of can	(1,100)	(340)
Potatoes:		
Cooked:		
Baked in skin	4*	503
Boiled in skin	3*	407
Boiled, pared before cooking	2*	285
French-fried	6*	853
Fried from raw	223	775
Hash-browned after holding overnight	288	475

*No salt added.

74

	SODIUM (MG PER 3.5 OZ OR 100 G)	POTASSIUM (MG PER 3.5 OZ OR 100 G)
Potatoes continued		
Mashed, milk added	301	261
Mashed, milk & table fat added	331	250
Scalloped & au gratin:		
With cheese	447	306
Without cheese	355	327
Canned:		
Solids & liquid	1*	250
Dehydrated mashed:		
Flakes without milk:		
Prepared, water, milk, table fat added	231	286
Granules without milk:		
Prepared, water, milk, table fat added	256	290
Granules with milk:		
Prepared, water, table fat added	234	335
Frozen:		
Diced, for hash-browning:		
Cooked, hash-browned	299	283
French-fried:		
Heated	4*	652
Mashed:		
Heated	359	215
Potato chips	NA†	1,130
Potato flour	34	1,588
Potato salad, from home recipe, made with:		
Cooked salad dressing, seasonings	528	319
Mayonnaise & French dressing, hard-cooked egg, seasonings	480	296
Potato sticks	NA†	1,130
Pretzels	1,680‡	130
Prunes:		
Dehydrated, nugget-type & pieces:		

*No salt added.
†Sodium content is variable and may be as high as 1,000 mg per 100 cm.
‡Sodium content is variable. For example, very thin pretzel sticks contain about twice the average amount listed.

	SODIUM (MG PER 3.5 OZ OR 100 G)	POTASSIUM (MG PER 3.5 OZ OR 100 G)
Prunes continued		
Cooked, fruit & liquid, with added sugar	4	329
Dried, "softenized":		
Uncooked	8	694
Cooked (fruit & liquid):		
Without added sugar	4	327
With added sugar	3	262
Prune juice, canned or bottled	2	235
Prune whip	164	290
Puddings, with starch base, prepared from home recipe:		
See also Bread; Rennin products; Rice pudding; Tapioca; Baby food.		
Chocolate	56	171
Vanilla (blanc mange)	65	138
Pumpkin, canned	2	240
Rabbit, domesticated, cooked, stewed	41	368
Radishes, raw, common	18	322
Raisins, natural (unbleached):		
Uncooked	27	763
Cooked, fruit & liquid, added sugar	13	355
Raspberries:		
Raw:		
Black	1	199
Red	1	168
Canned, solids & liquid, water pack, with or without artificial sweetener:		
Black	1	135
Red	1	114
Frozen, red, sweetened, not thawed	1	100
Rennin products:		
Tablet (salts, starch, rennin enzyme)	22,300	NA
Dessert, home-prepared with tablet	82	126
Desserts prepared from mixes:		
Chocolate:		
Dessert made with milk	52	125

	SODIUM (MG PER 3.5 OZ OR 100 G)	POTASSIUM (MG PER 3.5 OZ OR 100 G)
Rennin continued		
Other flavors:		
Dessert made with milk	46	128
Rhubarb:		
Cooked, added sugar	2	203
Frozen, sweetened:		
Cooked, added sugar	3	176
Rice:		
Brown:		
Cooked	282	70
White (fully milled or polished):		
Enriched:		
Common commercial varieties, all types:		
Cooked	374	28
Long-grain:		
Parboiled; cooked	358	43
Precooked; ready-to-serve	273	Trace
Unenriched:		
Common commercial varieties, all types:		
Cooked	374	28
Rice bran	Trace	1,495
Rice products used mainly as hot breakfast cereals:		
Rice, granulated, added nutrients:		
Cooked	176	Trace
Rice products used mainly as ready-to-eat breakfast cereals:		
Rice flakes; added nutrients	987	180
Rice, puffed; added nutrients, without salt	2	100
Rice, puffed or oven popped, presweetened:		
Honey & added nutrients	706	NA
Honey or cocoa & added nutrients, including fat	358	61
Rice, shredded; added nutrients	846	NA
Rice, with protein concentrate, mainly:		
Casein, other added nutrients	600	NA
Wheat gluten, other added nutrients	800	NA

	SODIUM (MG PER 3.5 OZ OR 100 G)	POTASSIUM (MG PER 3.5 OZ OR 100 G)
Rice pudding with raisins	71	177
Rockfish, including black, canary, yellowtail, rasphead & bocaccio:		
Cooked, oven-steamed (with onions)	68	446
Roe; cooked, baked or broiled, cod & shad (prepared with butter or margarine & lemon juice or vinegar)	73	132
Rolls & buns:		
Baked from home recipe, with milk & enriched flour	279	117
Commercial:		
Ready-to-serve:		
Danish pastry	366	112
Hard rolls:		
Enriched	625	97
Unenriched	625	97
Plain (pan rolls):		
Enriched	506	95
Unenriched	506	95
Raisin rolls or buns	384	245
Sweet rolls	389	124
Whole wheat rolls	564	292
Partially baked (brown-&-serve):		
Enriched:		
Unbrowned	513	91
Browned	562	100
Unenriched:		
Unbrowned	513	91
Browned	562	100
Rolls baked from roll dough:		
Enriched rolls, baked	560	96
Unenriched rolls, baked	560	96
Rolls baked from roll mix:		
Rolls made with water	313	123
Rusk	246	161
Rutabagas:		
Cooked, boiled, drained	4	167
Rye:		
Whole grain	(1)	467
Flours:		
Light	(1)	156

	SODIUM (MG PER 3.5 OZ OR 100 G)	POTASSIUM (MG PER 3.5 OZ OR 100 G)
Rye continued		
Medium	(1)	203
Dark	1	860
Rye wafers, whole grain	882	600
Safflower seed kernels, dry	NA	NA
Salad dressings, commercial:		
Blue & Roquefort cheese:		
Regular	1,094	37
Special dietary (low-calorie):		
Low-fat (approx. 5 cal. per tsp.)	1,108	34
Low-fat (approx. 1 cal. per tsp.)	1,134	29
French:		
Regular	1,370	79
Special dietary (low-calorie):		
Low-fat (approx. 5 cal. per tsp.)	787	79
Low-fat with artificial sweetener (approx. 1 cal. per tsp.)	787	79
Medium-fat with artificial sweetener (approx. 10 cal. per tsp.)	787	79
Italian:		
Regular	2,092	15
Special dietary (low-calorie, approx. 2 cal. per tsp.)	787	15
Mayonnaise	597	34
Russian	868	157
Salad dressing (Mayonnaise type):		
Regular	586	9
Special dietary (low-calorie, approx. 8 cal. per tsp.)	118	9
Thousand Island:		
Regular	700	113
Special dietary (low-calorie, approx. 10 cal. per tsp.)	700	113
Salad dressings, made from home recipe:		
French	659	26
Cooked	728	116

	SODIUM (MG PER 3.5 OZ OR 100 G)	POTASSIUM (MG PER 3.5 OZ OR 100 G)
Salmon:		
Atlantic; canned, solids & liquid	NA	NA
Chinook (king); canned, solids & liquid	45*	366
Chum; canned, solids & liquid	53*	336
Coho (silver); canned, solids & liquid	351*	339
Pink (humpback); canned, solids & liquid	387*	361
Sockeye (red); canned, solids & liquid	522*	344
Salmon, cooked, broiled or baked	116	443
Salmon rice loaf	NA	NA
Salmon, smoked	NA	NA
Salt, table	38,758	4
Salt, sticks:		
Regular type	1,674	92
Vienna bread type	1,565	94
Sandwich spread (with chopped pickle):		
Regular	626	92
Special dietary (low-calorie, approx. 5 cal. per tsp.)	626	92
Sardines, Atlantic, canned in oil:		
Drained solids	823	590
Sardines, Pacific:		
Canned:		
In brine or mustard, solids & liquid	760	260
In oil, drained solids	NA	NA
In tomato sauce, solids & liquid	400	320
Sauerkraut, canned, solids & liquid (salt content 1.9% in finished product)	747	140
Sauerkraut juice, canned (salt content 2.0% in finished product)	787	NA
Sausage, cold cuts & luncheon meats:		
Blood sausage or blood pudding	NA	NA
Bockwurst	NA	NA

*For product canned without salt.

	SODIUM (MG PER 3.5 OZ OR 100 G)	POTASSIUM (MG PER 3.5 OZ OR 100 G)
Sausage continued		
Bologna:		
All samples	1,300	230
All meat	NA	NA
With nonfat dry milk	NA	NA
With cereal	NA	NA
Braunschweiger	NA	NA
Brown-&-serve sausage	NA	NA
Capicola or Capacola	NA	NA
Cervelat	NA	NA
Country-style sausage	NA	NA
Deviled ham, canned	NA	NA
Frankfurters; all samples	1,100	220
Headcheese	NA	NA
Knockwurst	NA	NA
Liverwurst	NA	NA
Luncheon meat:		
Boiled ham	NA	NA
Pork, cured ham or shoulder, chopped, spiced or unspiced, canned	1,234	222
Meatloaf	NA	NA
Meat, potted (includes potted beef, chicken & turkey)	NA	NA
Minced ham	NA	NA
Mortadella	NA	NA
Polish-style sausage	NA	NA
Pork & beef (chopped together)	NA	NA
Pork sausage, links or bulk:		
Cooked	958	269
Pork sausage, canned, drained solids	NA	NA
Salami	NA	NA
Scrapple	NA	NA
Souse	NA	NA
Thuringer	NA	NA
Vienna Sausage, canned	NA	NA
Scallops, bay & sea:		
Cooked, steamed	265	476
Frozen, breaded, fried, reheated	NA	NA
Seaweed, raw (kelp)	3,007	5,273
Sesame seeds, dry:		
Whole	60	725
Decorticated	NA	NA

81

	SODIUM (MG PER 3.5 OZ OR 100 G)	POTASSIUM (MG PER 3.5 OZ OR 100 G)
Shad or American Shad:		
Cooked:		
Baked (prepared with butter or margarine & bacon slices)	79	377
Creole (prepared with tomatoes, onion, green pepper, butter, & flour)	73	280
Canned, solids & liquid	NA	NA
Shallot bulbs, raw	12	334
Sherbet, orange	10	22
Shrimp:		
Raw	140	220
Cooked, French-fried (dipped in egg, bread crumbs, & flour or in batter)	186	229
Canned:		
Wet pack, solids & liquid	NA	NA
Dry pack or drained solids of wet pack	NA	122
Frozen, breaded, raw; not more than 50% breading	NA	NA
Shrimp or lobster paste, canned	NA	NA
Smelt, Atlantic, jack & bay:		
Canned, solids & liquid	NA	NA
Soups, commercial:		
Canned:		
Asparagus, cream of:		
Condensed	820	100
Prepared with equal volume of water	410	50
Prepared with equal volume of milk	436	123
Bean with pork:		
Condensed	806	316
Prepared with equal volume of water	403	158
Beef broth, bouillon, & consomme:		
Condensed	652	108
Prepared with equal volume of water	326	54
Beef noodle:		
Condensed	764	64

	SODIUM (MG PER 3.5 OZ OR 100 G)	POTASSIUM (MG PER 3.5 OZ OR 100 G)
Soups continued		
Prepared with equal volume of water	382	32
Celery, cream of:		
Condensed	796	90
Prepared with equal volume of water	398	45
Prepared with equal volume of milk	424	118
Chicken consomme:		
Condensed	602	NA
Prepared with equal volume of water	301	NA
Chicken, cream of:		
Condensed	809	66
Prepared with equal volume of water	404	33
Prepared with equal volume of milk	430	106
Chicken gumbo:		
Condensed	792	89
Prepared with equal volume of water	396	45
Chicken noodle:		
Condensed	816	46
Prepared with equal volume of water	408	23
Chicken with rice:		
Condensed	764	82
Prepared with equal volume of water	382	41
Chicken vegetable:		
Condensed	845	80
Prepared with equal volume of water	422	40
Clam chowder, Manhattan type (with tomatoes, without milk):		
Condensed	766	150
Prepared with equal volume of water	383	75
Minestrone:		
Condensed	813	255

	SODIUM (MG PER 3.5 OZ OR 100 G)	POTASSIUM (MG PER 3.5 OZ OR 100 G)
Soup continued		
Prepared with equal volume of water	406	128
Mushroom, cream of:		
Condensed	795	82
Prepared with equal volume of water	398	41
Prepared with equal volume of milk	424	114
Onion:		
Condensed	875	86
Prepared with equal volume of water	438	43
Pea, green:		
Condensed	734	160
Prepared with equal volume of water	367	80
Prepared with equal volume of milk	393	153
Pea, split:		
Condensed	767	220
Prepared with equal volume of water	384	110
Tomato:		
Condensed	792	188
Prepared with equal volume of water	396	94
Prepared with equal volume of milk	422	167
Turkey noodle:		
Condensed	832	64
Prepared with equal volume of water	416	32
Vegetable beef:		
Condensed	854	131
Prepared with equal volume of water	427	66
Vegetable with beef broth:		
Condensed	690	196
Prepared with equal volume of water	345	98
Vegetarian vegetable:		
Condensed	684	140
Prepared with equal volume of water	342	70

	SODIUM (MG PER 3.5 OZ OR 100 G)	POTASSIUM (MG PER 3.5 OZ OR 100 G)
Soup continued		
Dehydrated:		
Beef noodle:		
Prepared with 2 oz mix in 3 cups water	175	17
Chicken noodle:		
Prepared with 2 oz mix in 4 cups water	241	8
Chicken rice:		
Prepared with 1½ oz mix in 3 cups water	259	4
Onion:		
Prepared with 1½ oz mix in 4 cups water	287	24
Pea, green:		
Prepared with 2 oz mix in 3 cups water	325	120
Tomato vegetable with noodles:		
Prepared with 2½ oz mix in 4 cups water	427	12
Frozen:		
Clam chowder, New England type (with milk, without tomatoes):		
Condensed	870	185
Prepared with equal volume of water	435	92
Prepared with equal volume of milk	461	166
Pea, green, with ham:		
Condensed	750	20
Prepared with equal volume of water	375	100
Potato, cream of:		
Condensed	980	185
Prepared with equal volume of water	490	92
Prepared with equal volume of milk	516	166
Shrimp, cream of:		
Condensed	860	48
Prepared with equal volume of water	430	24

	SODIUM (MG PER 3.5 OZ OR 100 G)	POTASSIUM (MG PER 3.5 OZ OR 100 G)
Soups continued		
Prepared with equal volume of milk	456	97
Vegetable with beef:		
Condensed	792	145
Prepared with equal volume of water	396	72
Soybeans:		
Immature seeds:		
Cooked, boiled, drained	NA	NA
Canned, drained solids	236*	NA
Mature seeds, dry:		
Cooked (unsalted)	2	540
Fermented products:		
Natto (soybeans)	NA	249
Miso (cereal & soybeans)	2,950	334
Sprouted seeds:		
Cooked, boiled, drained	NA	NA
Soybean curd (tofu)	7	42
Soybean flours:		
Full-fat	1	1,660
High-fat	1	1,775
Low-fat	1	1,859
Defatted	1	1,820
Soybean milk:		
Fluid	NA	NA
Powder	NA	NA
Soybean milk products, sweetened:		
Liquid concentrate	43	237
Powder	1	915
Soybean protein	210	180
Soybean proteinate	1,200	NA
Soy sauce	7,325	366
Spaghetti:		
Enriched:		
Cooked, firm stage, "al dente" (8–10 min.)	1	79
Cooked, tender stage (14–20 min.)	1	61
Unenriched:		
Cooked, firm stage, "al dente" (8–10 min.)	1	79

*Estimated average based on the addition of salt in the amount of 0.6 percent of the finished product.

	SODIUM (MG PER 3.5 OZ OR 100 G)	POTASSIUM (MG PER 3.5 OZ OR 100 G)
Spaghetti continued		
Cooked, tender stage (14–20 min.)	1	61
Spaghetti in tomato sauce with cheese:		
Cooked, from home recipe	(382)	163
Canned	382	121
Spaghetti with meatballs in tomato sauce:		
Cooked, from home recipe	407	268
Canned	488	98
Spanish rice, cooked from home recipe	316	231
Spinach:		
Raw	71	470
Cooked, boiled, drained	50	324
Canned:		
Regular pack:		
Drained solids	236*	250
Special dietary pack (low-sodium):		
Drained solids	32	250
Frozen:		
Chopped:		
Cooked, boiled, drained	52	333
Leaf:		
Cooked, boiled, drained	49	362
Squash:		
Summer:		
All varieties:		
Raw	1	202
Cooked, boiled, drained	1	141
Crook neck & straight neck, yellow:		
Raw	1	202
Cooked, boiled, drained	1	141
Scallop varieties, white & pale green:		
Raw	1	202
Cooked, boiled, drained	1	141
Zucchini & Cocozelle (Italian marrow type), green:		
Raw	1	202

*Estimated average based on the addition of salt in the amount of 0.6 percent of the finished product.

	SODIUM (MG PER 3.5 OZ OR 100 G)	POTASSIUM (MG PER 3.5 OZ OR 100 G)
Squash continued		
Cooked, boiled, drained	1	141
Winter:		
All varieties:		
Raw	1	369
Cooked:		
Baked	1	461
Boiled, mashed	1	258
Acorn:		
Raw	1	384
Cooked:		
Baked	1	480
Boiled, mashed	1	269
Butternut:		
Raw	1	487
Cooked:		
Baked	1	609
Boiled, mashed	1	341
Hubbarb:		
Raw	1	217
Cooked:		
Baked	1	271
Boiled, mashed	1	152
Squash, frozen:		
Summer, yellow crook neck:		
Not thawed	3	167
Cooked, boiled, drained	3	167
Winter:		
Not thawed	1	207
Heated	1	207
Strawberries:		
Raw	1	164
Canned, solids & liquid:		
Water pack, with or without		
artificial sweetener	1	111
Frozen, sweetened, not thawed:		
Sliced	1	112
Whole	1	104
Sturgeon:		
Cooked, steamed	108	235
Smoked	NA	NA

	SODIUM (MG PER 3.5 OZ OR 100 G)	POTASSIUM (MG PER 3.5 OZ OR 100 G)
Succotash (corn & lima beans), frozen:		
Cooked, boiled, drained	38	246
Sugars:		
Beet or cane:		
Brown	30	344
Granulated	1	3
Powdered	1	3
Dextrose:		
Anhydrous	NA	NA
Crystallized	NA	NA
Maple	14	242
Sunflower seed kernels, dry	30	920
Sweetbreads (thymus):		
Beef (yearlings):		
Cooked, braised	116	433
Calf:		
Cooked, braised	NA	NA
Lamb:		
Cooked, braised	NA	NA
Sweet potatoes:		
Cooked, all:		
Baked in skin	12	300
Boiled in skin	10	243
Candied	42	190
Canned:		
Liquid pack, solids & liquid:		
Regular pack in syrup	48	(120)
Special dietary pack, without added sugar & salt	12	120
Vacuum or solid pack:		
Regular pack	48	200
Special dietary pack (low-sodium)	12	200
Dehydrated flakes:		
Prepared with water	45	140
Swordfish, cooked, broiled (prepared with butter or margarine)	NA	NA
Syrups:		
Cane	NA	425
Maple	10	176

	SODIUM (MG PER 3.5 OZ OR 100 G)	POTASSIUM (MG PER 3.5 OZ OR 100 G)
Syrups continued		
Sorghum	NA	NA
Table blends:		
Chiefly corn, light & dark	68	4
Cane & maple	2	26
Tangerine juice:		
Raw (Dancy variety)	1	178
Canned:		
Unsweetened	1	178
Sweetened	1	178
Frozen concentrate, unsweetened:		
Undiluted	2	613
Diluted with 3 parts water, by volume	1	174
Tapioca desserts:		
Apple tapioca	51	26
Tapioca cream pudding	156	135
Tartar sauce:		
Regular	707	78
Special dietary (low-calorie, approx. 10 cal. per tsp.)	707	78
Tea, instant (water-soluble solids) carbohydrate added:		
Dry powder	NA	4,530
Beverage	NA	25
Tilefish:		
Cooked, baked	NA	NA
Tomatoes, ripe:		
Raw	3	244
Cooked, boiled	4	287
Canned, solids & liquid:		
Regular pack	130	217
Special dietary pack (low sodium)	3	217
Tomato catsup, bottled	1,042*	363
Tomato chili sauce, bottled	1,338*	(370)
Tomato juice:		
Canned or bottled:		
Regular pack	200	227
Special dietary pack (low-sodium)	3	227

*Applies to regular pack. For special dietary pack (low-sodium), values range from 5 to 35 mg per 100 gms.

	SODIUM (MG PER 3.5 OZ OR 100 G)	POTASSIUM (MG PER 3.5 OZ OR 100 G)
Tomatoes continued		
Canned concentrate:		
Diluted with 3 parts water, by volume	209	235
Dehydrated (crystals):		
Prepared with water (1 lb. yields approx. 1¾ gals.)	(258)	231
Tomato juice cocktail, canned or bottled	200	221
Tomato paste, canned (no salt added)	38*	888
Tomato puree, canned:		
Regular pack	399	426
Special dietary pack (low-sodium)	6	426
Tongue:		
Beef:		
Medium-fat:		
Cooked, braised	61	164
Thin (very thin), raw	NA	NA
Smoked	NA	NA
Calf:		
Cooked, braised	NA	NA
Hog:		
Cooked, braised	NA	NA
Lamb:		
Cooked, braised	NA	NA
Sheep:		
Cooked, braised	NA	NA
Tongue, canned or cured (beef, lamb, etc.):		
Whole, canned or pickled	NA	NA
Potted or deviled	NA	NA
Tripe, beef, pickled	46	19
Trout, rainbow or steelhead, canned	NA	NA
Tuna:		
Raw:		
Bluefin	NA	NA
Yellowfin	37†	NA

*If salt is added, the sodium content is about 790 mg per 100 gm.
†One sample contained 439 mg of sodium per 100 gm.

	SODIUM (MG PER 3.5 OZ OR 100 G)	POTASSIUM (MG PER 3.5 OZ OR 100 G)
Tuna continued		
Canned:		
In oil:		
Drained solids	533	200
In water:		
Solids & liquid	41*	270*
Tuna salad (prepared with tuna, celery, pickle, mayonnaise, onion, & egg)	NA	NA
Turkey:		
All classes:		
Total edible:		
Cooked, roasted	NA	NA
Flesh & skin:		
Cooked, roasted	NA	NA
Flesh only:		
Cooked, roasted	130	367
Light meat:		
Cooked, roasted	82	411
Dark meat:		
Cooked, roasted	99	398
Turkey, canned, meat only	NA	NA
Turkey pot pie:		
Home-prepared, baked	273	198
Commercial, frozen, unheated	369	114
Turnips, cooked, boiled, drained	34	188
Turnip greens, leaves, including stems:		
Cooked, boiled, drained, cooked in:		
Small amount of water, short time	NA	NA
Large amount of water, long time	NA	NA
Canned, solids & liquid	236†	243
Frozen:		
Cooked, boiled, drained	17	149

*One sample with salt added contained 875 mg of sodium per 100 gm and 275 mg of potassium.
†Estimated average based on the addition of salt in the amount of 0.6 percent of the finished product.

	SODIUM (MG PER 3.5 OZ OR 100 G)	POTASSIUM (MG PER 3.5 OZ OR 100 G)
Turtle, green, canned	NA	NA
Veal:		
Retail cuts, untrimmed:		
Chuck:		
Medium-fat class:		
Cooked, braised	80	500
Flank:		
Medium-fat class:		
Cooked, stewed	80	500
Foreshank:		
Medium-fat class:		
Cooked, stewed	80	50
Loin:		
Medium-fat class:		
Cooked, broiled	80	500
Plate:		
Medium-fat class:		
Cooked, stewed	80	500
Rib:		
Medium-fat class:		
Cooked, roasted	80	500
Round with rump:		
Medium-fat class:		
Cooked, broiled	80	500
Vegetable juice cocktail, canned	(200)	(221)
Vegetable main dishes, canned:		
Principal ingredients:		
Peanuts & soya	NA	NA
Wheat protein	NA	NA
Wheat protein, nuts or peanuts	NA	NA
Wheat protein, vegetable oil	NA	NA
Wheat & soy protein	NA	NA
Wheat & soy protein, soy or other vegetable oil	NA	NA
Vegetables, mixed (carrots, corn, peas, green snap beans, lima beans), frozen:		
Cooked, boiled, drained	53	191
Vinegar:		
Cider	1	100
Distilled	1	15

	SODIUM (MG PER 3.5 OZ OR 100 G)	POTASSIUM (MG PER 3.5 OZ OR 100 G)
Waffles:		
Baked from home recipe, made with:		
Enriched flour	475	145
Unenriched flour	475	145
Waffles baked from waffle mixes:		
Waffles, made with water (enriched or unenriched flour)	560	55
Waffles & pancakes, made with egg, milk (enriched or unenriched flour used in the mix)	686	195
Walnuts:		
Black	3	460
Persian or English	2	450
Waterchestnut, Chinese (matai, waternut), raw	20	500
Watercress leaves including stems, raw	52	282
Watermelon, raw	1	100
Weakfish, cooked, broiled (salt added in cooking)	560	465
Welsh rarebit	332	138
Wheat flours:		
Whole (from hard wheats)	3	370
Patent:		
All-purpose or family flour:		
Enriched	2	95
Unenriched	2	95
Bread flour:		
Enriched	2	95
Unenriched	2	95
Cake or pastry flour	2	95
Gluten flour	2	60
Self-rising flour, enriched (anhydrous monocalcium phosphate used as a baking acid)*	1,079	90

*The acid ingredient most commonly used in self-rising flour. When sodium acid pyrophosphate in combination with either anhydrous monocalcium phosphate or calcium carbonate is used, the value for sodium is 1,360 mg.

	SODIUM (MG PER 3.5 OZ OR 100 G)	POTASSIUM (MG PER 3.5 OZ OR 100 G)
Wheat bran, crude, commercially milled	9	1,121
Wheat germ, crude, commercially milled	3	827
Wheat products used mainly as hot breakfast cereals:		
Wheat, rolled:		
Cooked	295	84
Wheat, whole-meal:		
Cooked	212	48
Wheat & malted barley cereal, toasted:		
Quick-cooking:		
Cooked	72	Trace
Instant-cooking:		
Cooked	102	Trace
Wheat products used mainly as ready-to-eat breakfast cereals:		
Wheat flakes, added nutrients	1,032	NA
Wheat germ, toasted	2	947
Wheat, puffed:		
Added nutrients, without salt	4	340
Added nutrients (including salt), with sugar & honey	161	99
Wheat, shredded:		
Without salt or other added ingredients	3	348
With malt, salt, & sugar added	697	NA
Wheat & malted barley flakes, nutrients added	780	NA
Wheat & malted barley granules, nutrients added	710	23
Whey, fluid	NA	NA
Whitefish, lake:		
Cooked, baked, stuffed (prepared with bacon, butter, onion, celery & bread crumbs)	195	291
Smoked	NA	NA
White Sauce:		
Thin	351	146
Medium	379	139
Thick	399	133

	SODIUM (MG PER 3.5 OZ OR 100 G)	POTASSIUM (MG PER 3.5 OZ OR 100 G)
Wild rice, raw	7	220
Yogurt:		
Made from partially skimmed milk	51	143
Made from whole milk	47	132
Zwieback	250	150